Intermittent Fasting
for beginners

A Guide to Weight Loss Using
Intermittent Fasting For both men
and women

By

Vanessa Owens

Table of content

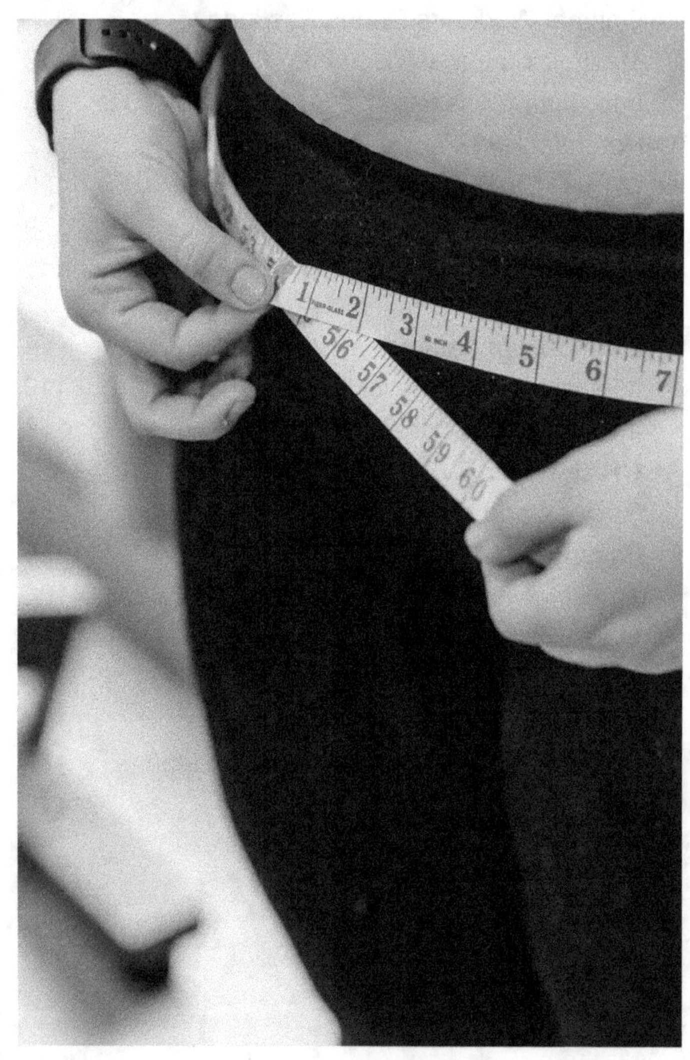

Introduction

In the fast-paced realm of contemporary living, where time is a precious commodity and wellness often takes a back seat to the demands of daily life, Vanessa Owens emerges as a protagonist navigating the delicate balance between career, health, and self-discovery. With an inquisitive spirit and a fervent desire for holistic well-being, Vanessa embarks on a transformative journey into the world of intermittent fasting, an uncharted territory within the bustling landscape of modern lifestyles.

Vanessa's tale unfolds against the backdrop of her urban existence, where the relentless tick-tock of the clock mirrors the perpetual rhythm of city life. Faced with the challenges of a demanding career and the constant barrage of information on health and diet trends, Vanessa stumbles upon intermittent fasting as a beacon of hope, a potential solution to the tumultuous equation of work-life equilibrium.

As the author of her narrative, Vanessa shares her intimate experiences, demystifying the intricacies of intermittent fasting. Her journey becomes a narrative bridge for readers seeking not only physical transformation but a profound reconnection with their bodies and a recalibration of their relationship with food. Through Vanessa's lens, intermittent fasting evolves from a mere dietary strategy to a lifestyle philosophy—one that challenges societal norms and empowers individuals to take charge of their well-being.

The introductory chapters set the stage, inviting readers to join Vanessa in her exploration of different fasting protocols, scientific underpinnings, and the art of mindful nourishment. It's a tale of self-discovery, resilience, and the pursuit of a more meaningful and sustainable approach to health in an age where time feels elusive, and well-being is a coveted treasure. Vanessa's journey promises not just a guide to intermittent fasting but a testament to the potential for transformative change within the confines of a time-pressed, modern existence.

CHAPTER ONE

Understanding Intermittent Fasting

Intermittent fasting (IF) is a dietary approach that alternates between periods of eating and fasting, offering a unique perspective on when, rather than what, we eat. At its core, IF harnesses the body's natural ability to adapt to periods of food scarcity, triggering a cascade of physiological changes with numerous health implications.

The physiological effects of intermittent fasting are multifaceted. During fasting periods, insulin levels drop, prompting the body to shift from utilizing glucose to burning stored fat for energy. This metabolic switch not only facilitates weight loss but also activates cellular repair mechanisms like autophagy. This process involves the removal of damaged cellular components, contributing to improved overall cellular health.

There are various methods of intermittent fasting, each with its own unique approach. Time-restricted eating (TRE) involves limiting daily food intake to a specific time window, such as 16 hours of fasting followed by an 8-hour eating window. Alternate-day fasting, 5:2 fasting, and the Warrior Diet are other popular variations that introduce intermittent calorie restriction on specific days or times.

Beyond weight management, intermittent fasting has been associated with improved metabolic health. It enhances insulin sensitivity, reducing the risk of type 2 diabetes, and may positively influence cardiovascular health markers. Additionally, intermittent fasting has shown potential cognitive benefits, including increased focus and neuroprotective effects.

Getting started with intermittent fasting involves selecting a method aligned with individual preferences, gradually adjusting to fasting periods, and dispelling common misconceptions. Practical tips for success include mindful meal planning, staying hydrated during fasting windows, incorporating regular exercise, and effectively managing hunger cues.

While intermittent fasting has demonstrated significant benefits, it's essential to consider individual variations and potential risks. Consulting with healthcare professionals, addressing nutrient concerns, and navigating social aspects are crucial components for a sustainable intermittent fasting journey. By understanding the underlying principles, embracing flexibility, and incorporating intermittent fasting into a holistic lifestyle, individuals can unlock a powerful tool for improved health and well-being.

Brief History and Evolutionary Context of Intermittent Fasting

- ## Historical Roots:

Intermittent fasting (IF) traces its roots back to ancient cultures and religious practices. Fasting has been a part of human history for millennia, often associated with spiritual rituals and rites of passage. In various religions, fasting has been observed as a means of purification, self-discipline, and spiritual reflection.

- ## Evolutionary Perspective:

From an evolutionary standpoint, intermittent fasting aligns with our ancestors' eating patterns. Hunter-gatherer societies experienced periods of feast and famine due to the unpredictability of food availability. Our bodies evolved mechanisms to thrive in these conditions, with the ability to efficiently store energy during times of plenty and tap into stored reserves during scarcity.

- **Early Observations:**

The concept of intermittent fasting gained attention in the early 20th century when researchers observed health benefits associated with caloric restriction. In the 1930s, experiments with rodents demonstrated that restricting calorie intake without malnutrition extended lifespan, sparking interest in the broader implications of fasting on health.

- **Research and Scientific Exploration:**

The 21st century witnessed a resurgence of interest in intermittent fasting, fueled by advances in scientific research. Studies began exploring the metabolic and cellular responses to periods of fasting, shedding light on the potential benefits for weight management, metabolic health, and longevity.

- ## Popularization in the 21st Century:

In recent decades, books, documentaries, and influential figures in the health and wellness industry have popularized intermittent fasting. Various methods, such as the 16/8 method, 5:2 fasting, and alternate-day fasting, gained prominence as individuals sought effective and sustainable approaches to weight loss and overall well-being.

- ## Clinical Applications and Medical Recognition:

Intermittent fasting moved beyond popular culture and gained recognition in medical and scientific circles. Research studies started investigating its impact on conditions like obesity, diabetes, and cardiovascular health. Some medical professionals began incorporating intermittent fasting as a complementary approach in patient care.

- ## Ongoing Exploration and Future Directions:

As of the knowledge cutoff in 2022, ongoing research continues to unravel the physiological mechanisms and potential applications of intermittent fasting. Scientists explore its effects on aging, cognitive function, and various disease states. The field is dynamic, with emerging studies contributing to a deeper understanding of how intermittent fasting can positively influence human health.

Intermittent fasting, rooted in historical practices and reflecting our evolutionary adaptations, has evolved from traditional rituals to a scientifically explored and increasingly recognized approach to health and wellness. Its journey from ancient traditions to mainstream recognition underscores the enduring human fascination with optimizing well-being through mindful eating patterns. As research progresses, intermittent fasting remains an intriguing field with the potential to shape the future of dietary recommendations and lifestyle interventions.

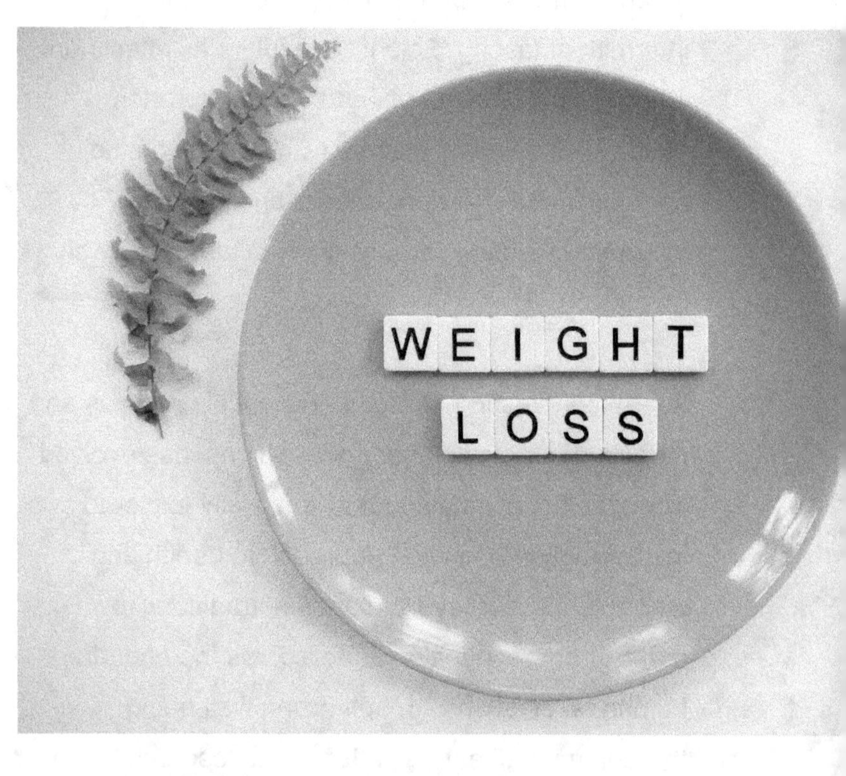

WEIGHT
LOSS

CHAPTER TWO

Benefits of Intermittent Fasting

• Weight Management:

Intermittent fasting is widely recognized for its effectiveness in weight management. By creating a controlled eating window, individuals naturally consume fewer calories, leading to weight loss. Additionally, the metabolic switch to burning stored fat during fasting periods contributes to fat loss while preserving lean muscle mass.

- ## Improved Metabolic Health:

IF has shown positive effects on metabolic health by enhancing insulin sensitivity. This can lower the risk of developing insulin resistance and type 2 diabetes. Fasting periods also contribute to better blood sugar control, promoting overall metabolic well-being.

- ## Cellular Repair and Autophagy:

Fasting triggers autophagy, a cellular process where the body cleans out damaged cells and regenerates new, healthy ones. This contributes to improved cellular repair mechanisms, potentially reducing the risk of various diseases and promoting longevity.

- ## Cardiovascular Health:

Intermittent fasting may have cardiovascular benefits, including reduced blood pressure, improved cholesterol levels, and enhanced heart health. These factors contribute to a lower risk of heart disease and related complications.

- ## Cognitive Benefits:

Some studies suggest that intermittent fasting may positively impact cognitive function. Improved brain health, increased production of brain-derived neurotrophic factor (BDNF), and reduced oxidative stress are potential mechanisms that contribute to enhanced cognitive performance.

- ## Longevity and Aging:

Research on animal models indicates that intermittent fasting may extend lifespan and promote longevity. While the direct translation to humans is still under investigation, the cellular repair processes activated during fasting could potentially slow down the aging process.

- ## Inflammation Reduction:

IF has been associated with reduced inflammation markers in the body. Chronic inflammation is linked to various health issues, including autoimmune

diseases and certain cancers. By mitigating
inflammation, intermittent fasting may contribute to
overall well-being.

- ## Enhanced Fat Oxidation and Ketosis:

During fasting periods, the body shifts to fat
oxidation for energy, leading to the production of
ketone bodies. This state of ketosis has been linked
to improved energy levels, mental clarity, and
metabolic flexibility.

- ## Hormonal Regulation:

Intermittent fasting influences the secretion of
hormones such as growth hormone and
norepinephrine. Increased growth hormone levels
contribute to muscle preservation and fat utilization,
while elevated norepinephrine enhances metabolic
rate.

- ## Simplicity and Flexibility:

One notable benefit of intermittent fasting is its
simplicity and flexibility. It doesn't require intricate
meal planning or complex dietary restrictions.
Individuals can choose a fasting method that suits
their lifestyle, making it a sustainable approach for
many.

While intermittent fasting offers various benefits, it's
crucial to note that individual responses can vary.
Consulting with healthcare professionals before
adopting a fasting regimen, especially for individuals
with pre-existing health conditions, is advisable.
Overall, the diverse array of advantages associated
with intermittent fasting continues to fuel its
popularity as a holistic approach to health and
well-being.

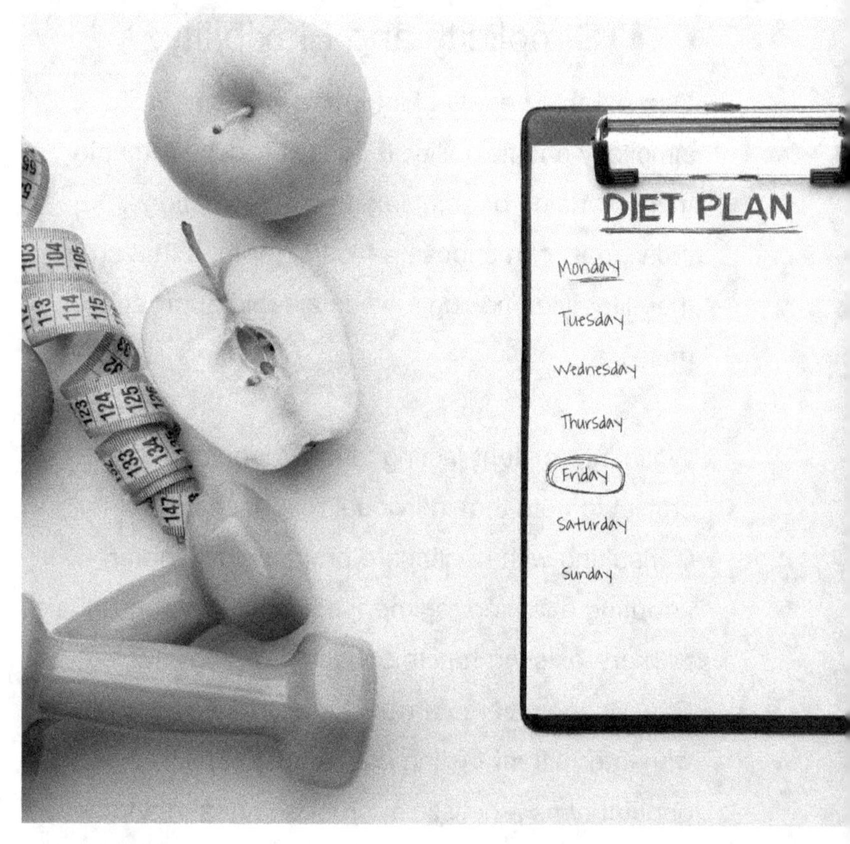
DIET PLAN
Monday
Tuesday
Wednesday
Thursday
Friday
Saturday
Sunday

CHAPTER THREE

Different Intermittent Fasting Method

❖ Time-Restricted Eating (TRE):

- *Methodology*: Involves limiting daily food intake to a specific time window and fasting for the remaining hours. For example, the 16/8 method consists of a daily 16-hour fast followed by an 8-hour eating window.

- *Benefits*: Simplicity and ease of implementation make this method popular. It aligns with the body's natural circadian rhythms, potentially optimizing metabolic processes.

Time-Restricted Eating (TRE) is a dietary approach that involves limiting the time window during which one consumes food. The primary focus of TRE is not on what you eat but rather when you eat it. This concept is rooted in the idea that aligning eating patterns with natural circadian rhythms can positively impact metabolic health.

Key Principles:

- *Time Window*:

TRE typically involves a daily time window for eating, such as an 8- to 12-hour period. For example, if someone follows a 10-hour TRE, they might consume all their daily meals within a 10-hour timeframe and abstain from caloric intake for the remaining 14 hours.

- *Circadian Rhythms:*

The human body operates on a circadian rhythm, a 24-hour cycle influenced by environmental cues like light and darkness. TRE aims to synchronize eating patterns with these natural rhythms, suggesting that certain metabolic processes are optimized during specific times of the day.

- *Fasting Period:*

The fasting period during TRE is not necessarily an absolute fast from all nutrients. It commonly involves abstaining from caloric intake, but water, herbal teas, and black coffee are often allowed during the fasting window.

Potential Benefits:

- *Weight Management:* Some studies suggest that TRE may aid in weight management by promoting a more efficient use of nutrients and improving metabolic flexibility.

- *Blood Sugar Control:* TRE has been associated with improved insulin sensitivity, potentially reducing the risk of type 2 diabetes.

- *Cellular Repair and Longevity:* Fasting periods may stimulate autophagy, a cellular repair process. Some researchers propose that intermittent fasting, including TRE, might have implications for longevity.

- *Improved Sleep:* Aligning eating patterns with circadian rhythms may positively impact sleep quality, as digestion and metabolism are less active during the body's natural rest phase.

Considerations

- *Individual Variability:*

The effectiveness of TRE can vary among individuals. Factors such as lifestyle, health conditions, and personal preferences play a role.

- *Nutrient Intake:*

While TRE focuses on when to eat, it's crucial to maintain a balanced and nutrient-dense diet during the eating window to meet nutritional needs.

- *Consultation with Healthcare Professionals:*

Before adopting any dietary changes, especially if you have existing health conditions, it's advisable to consult with healthcare professionals or registered dietitians.

Time-Restricted Eating is a concept that continues to garner interest in the field of nutrition and health. While some research suggests potential benefits, more studies are needed to fully understand the long-term effects and individual variations. As with any dietary approach, it's essential to approach TRE with awareness, taking into account personal health goals and consulting with professionals when necessary.

❖ Alternate-Day Fasting:

- *Methodology:*

Alternates between days of regular eating and days of significant calorie reduction or complete fasting. This can involve consuming very few calories on fasting days.

- Benefits:

Can be effective for weight loss and offers flexibility. However, adherence might be challenging for some due to the alternating nature of eating patterns.

Alternate-Day Fasting (ADF) is a form of intermittent fasting that alternates between days of regular eating and days of significant caloric restriction or complete fasting. This dietary approach has gained attention for its potential benefits on weight management and metabolic health.

Key Principles

- *Fasting Days:*

On fasting days, individuals typically consume a very low amount of calories or abstain from caloric intake altogether. Some variations allow for a minimal caloric intake, often around 25% of daily energy needs.

- *Feeding Days:*

On non-fasting or feeding days, individuals eat freely, without specific restrictions on the types of food. It's important to note that these days are not characterized by overeating to compensate for the fasting days.

- *Intermittent Nature:*

ADF is considered a type of intermittent fasting because it cycles between periods of eating and fasting. This cyclical pattern is believed to provide metabolic benefits without continuous caloric restriction.

Potential Benefits

- *Weight Loss:*

ADF may lead to calorie reduction over time, contributing to weight loss. The intermittent nature of fasting may help individuals adhere to the plan compared to more traditional continuous caloric restriction.

- *Improved Insulin Sensitivity:*

Some studies suggest that ADF may improve insulin sensitivity, which is crucial for blood sugar control and may reduce the risk of type 2 diabetes.

- *Cardiometabolic Health:*

ADF has been associated with positive changes in cardiovascular health markers, such as improved lipid profiles and reduced blood pressure in some individuals.

- *Cellular Repair:*

Fasting periods in ADF may trigger autophagy, a cellular process that removes damaged cells and promotes cellular repair.

Considerations

- *Individual Variability:*

The effectiveness of ADF can vary among

individuals, and not everyone may find it sustainable

or suitable for their lifestyle.

- *Nutrient Intake:*

While ADF doesn't impose specific restrictions on

food choices, it's essential to focus on

nutrient-dense foods to meet nutritional needs on

feeding days.

- *Hydration:*

Staying adequately hydrated is crucial, especially on

fasting days. Water, herbal teas, and black coffee

are typically allowed during fasting periods.

- *Medical Considerations:*

Individuals with existing health conditions or those

taking medications should consult with healthcare

professionals before adopting ADF to ensure it is safe for them.

Alternate-Day Fasting is a form of intermittent fasting that holds promise for weight management and metabolic health. While some studies suggest potential benefits, more research is needed to fully understand the long-term effects and individual variations. As with any dietary approach, it's crucial to approach ADF with awareness, considering personal health goals and consulting with professionals when necessary.

❖ 5:2 Fasting:

- *Methodology:* Involves eating normally for five days a week and significantly restricting calorie intake (typically around 500-600 calories) on two non-consecutive days.

- *Benefits:* Provides a structured approach with clear fasting and non-fasting days. This method allows for some flexibility in choosing fasting days.

Fasting in intermittent fasting is a key component of this dietary approach, offering various potential health benefits. However, it's essential to approach intermittent fasting with awareness, understanding individual needs, and consulting with healthcare professionals when necessary. As with any lifestyle change, moderation and consistency are key factors for long-term success.

❖ Warrior Diet

- *Methodology:* Consists of a 20-hour daily fast followed by a 4-hour eating window in the evening. During the fasting period, small amounts of raw fruits and vegetables may be consumed.

- *Benefits:* Emphasizes undereating during the day and feasting in the evening. It may suit those who prefer a single large meal at night.

The Warrior Diet is a form of intermittent fasting that follows an eating pattern based on the presumed dietary habits of ancient warriors. Created by fitness expert Ori Hofmekler, this diet involves alternating between short periods of undereating or fasting during the day and a single large meal at night. The Warrior Diet places a strong emphasis on aligning eating patterns with the body's natural circadian rhythms.

Key Principles of the Warrior Diet

- *20/4 Eating Pattern:*
The Warrior Diet typically involves a daily fasting period of 20 hours, during which individuals consume small amounts of raw fruits and vegetables, and a 4-hour eating window in the evening for one large, nutrient-dense meal.

- *Undereating During the Day:*
The undereating phase encourages the consumption of low-calorie, nutrient-dense foods such as raw fruits, vegetables, and small amounts of protein.

- *Feasting at Night:*
The main meal, often referred to as the "feasting" phase, is characterized by consuming larger portions of proteins, carbohydrates, and healthy fats.

- *Circadian Rhythms:*

The Warrior Diet is designed to synchronize eating patterns with the body's circadian rhythms, with the undereating phase aligning with the natural slowdown of metabolism during the day and the feasting phase taking advantage of the body's ability to digest and absorb nutrients more efficiently in the evening.

Potential Benefits of the Warrior Diet

- *Weight Management:*

The caloric restriction during the undereating phase may contribute to overall calorie reduction, potentially aiding in weight management.

- *Improved Insulin Sensitivity:*

Fasting periods may enhance insulin sensitivity, supporting blood sugar control and reducing the risk of insulin resistance.

- *Promotion of Autophagy:*

Extended fasting periods, as seen in the Warrior Diet, may stimulate autophagy, a cellular repair process that removes damaged cells and promotes overall cellular health.

- *Increased Growth Hormone Production:*

Some proponents of the Warrior Diet suggest that the fasting period may lead to an increase in growth hormone production, potentially influencing muscle preservation and fat burning.

Considerations

- *Individual Adaptation:*

The Warrior Diet may not be suitable for everyone, and individual responses to this eating pattern can vary. It is crucial to actively listen to your body and make the necessary adjustments.

- *Nutrient Intake:*

During the feasting phase, it's crucial to focus on nutrient-dense foods to meet the body's nutritional needs adequately.

- *Hydration:*

Staying hydrated is important, and water consumption is encouraged during the undereating and feasting phases.

- *Professional Guidance:*

Individuals with existing health conditions, pregnant or breastfeeding women, and athletes should seek professional advice before adopting the Warrior Diet.

The Warrior Diet is a specific form of intermittent fasting that emphasizes undereating during the day and feasting at night. While some people may find benefits in terms of weight management and metabolic health, it's essential to approach this eating pattern with awareness, considering individual needs and consulting with healthcare professionals when necessary. As with any dietary approach, moderation and balance are key factors for long-term success.

❖ Eat-Stop-Eat:

- *Methodology:* Involves 24-hour fasts once or twice a week. This method requires a full day of fasting, typically from dinner one day to dinner the next day.

   - *Benefits:* Simplifies the fasting routine to one or two days a week, providing a break from continuous calorie intake.

Eat-Stop-Eat is a form of intermittent fasting characterized by a cycle of regular eating followed by extended periods of fasting. Created by fitness expert Brad Pilon, this approach involves fasting for a complete 24 hours once or twice a week. The primary focus of Eat-Stop-Eat is on the duration of the fasting period, allowing the body to experience a prolonged state without caloric intake.

Key Principles of Eat-Stop-Eat
- *24-Hour Fasting:*
The central component of Eat-Stop-Eat is a 24-hour fasting period. This usually involves abstaining from caloric intake from dinner one day to dinner the next day.

- *Frequency:*

Individuals following the Eat-Stop-Eat protocol may choose to implement it once or twice a week, depending on their preferences and lifestyle.

- *Flexibility:*

Eat-Stop-Eat allows for flexibility in food choices during non-fasting days, emphasizing that individuals can eat a regular, balanced diet when not fasting.

- *Hydration:*

Staying well-hydrated is crucial during the fasting period. Water, herbal teas, and black coffee are typically allowed and encouraged.

Potential Benefits of Eat-Stop-Eat

- *Weight Management:*

The extended fasting period in Eat-Stop-Eat may lead to a reduction in overall calorie intake, potentially contributing to weight loss over time.

- *Improved Insulin Sensitivity:*

Intermittent fasting has been associated with improved insulin sensitivity, which is beneficial for blood sugar control and may reduce the risk of type 2 diabetes.

- *Metabolic Adaptations:*
Fasting periods may induce metabolic adaptations, such as increased fat oxidation, which can contribute to fat loss.

- *Simplicity and Convenience:*
Eat-Stop-Eat can be relatively straightforward to implement as it doesn't require daily tracking of eating windows. This simplicity may make it more sustainable for some individuals.

Considerations

- *Individual Adaptation:*
The effectiveness and comfort of the Eat-Stop-Eat approach can vary among individuals. It may take time for the body to adapt to the fasting period, and individuals should pay attention to their own responses.

- *Nutrient Intake:*

While fasting, it's important to focus on nutrient-dense foods during non-fasting days to ensure that the body receives essential vitamins and minerals.

- *Professional Guidance:*
Individuals with existing health conditions, pregnant or breastfeeding women, and athletes should seek professional advice before adopting Eat-Stop-Eat.

- *Psychological Factors:*
Extended fasting periods may not be suitable for everyone, and individuals should consider their own psychological well-being and relationship with food.

Eat-Stop-Eat is an intermittent fasting approach that involves 24-hour fasting periods once or twice a week. While it may offer benefits in terms of weight management and metabolic health, individuals should approach this method with awareness, considering their own needs and consulting with healthcare professionals when necessary. As with any dietary approach, moderation, balance, and individualization are crucial for long-term success.

❖ OMAD (One Meal A Day)

- *Methodology:* Restricts eating to a single meal within a short time frame, usually a one-hour window. The remaining 23 hours of the day involve fasting.

- *Benefits:* Offers simplicity and may suit those who prefer fewer, larger meals. However, ensuring adequate nutrient intake within one meal is crucial.

One Meal a Day (OMAD) is a form of intermittent fasting characterized by a daily eating pattern that involves consuming all of one's daily caloric intake in a single meal, typically within a one-hour eating window. OMAD has gained popularity for its simplicity and potential health benefits, and it falls under the broader category of time-restricted eating.

Key Principles of OMAD
- *Extended Fasting Period:*

OMAD involves an extended fasting period, typically lasting 23 hours or more, followed by a short eating window of one hour.

- *Meal Composition:*

During the one-hour eating window, individuals consume a single, large meal that is intended to provide all the necessary nutrients and energy for the day.

- *Flexibility:*

While OMAD traditionally involves a 23:1 fasting-to-eating ratio, some variations may allow for a slightly longer eating window, such as a 22:2 or 20:4 ratio, depending on individual preferences.

- *Hydration:*

Staying well-hydrated is essential during the fasting period. Water, herbal teas, and black coffee are typically allowed and encouraged.

Potential Benefits of OMAD

- *Weight Management:*

OMAD can lead to a reduction in overall calorie intake, potentially contributing to weight loss. The extended fasting period may also promote fat utilization for energy.

- *Improved Insulin Sensitivity:*
Intermittent fasting, including OMAD, has been associated with improved insulin sensitivity, which is beneficial for blood sugar control.

- *Simplicity and Convenience:*
OMAD is relatively simple to follow, as it eliminates the need for multiple meals and snacks throughout the day. This simplicity may make it more sustainable for some individuals.

- *Potential Autophagy:*
The prolonged fasting period in OMAD may stimulate autophagy, a cellular repair process that removes damaged cells and supports overall cellular health.

Considerations
- *Individual Adaptation:*

OMAD may not be suitable for everyone, and individual responses can vary. Some individuals may find it challenging to adapt to the extended fasting period.

- *Nutrient Intake:*

It's crucial to ensure that the single meal consumed during the eating window is nutritionally balanced and provides all essential nutrients.

- *Professional Guidance:*

Individuals with existing health conditions, pregnant or breastfeeding women, and athletes should seek professional advice before adopting OMAD.

- Psychological Factors:

OMAD may impact individuals psychologically, especially those with a history of disordered eating. It's important to consider one's relationship with food and overall well-being.

OMAD is a specific form of intermittent fasting that involves consuming all daily calories in a single meal within a one-hour eating window. While it may offer benefits in terms of weight management and metabolic health, individuals should approach OMAD with awareness, considering their own needs and consulting with healthcare professionals when necessary. As with any dietary approach, moderation, balance, and individualization are crucial for long-term success.

❖ Spontaneous Meal Skipping

- *Methodology:* Involves occasional skipping of meals without a structured fasting plan. This can be spontaneous, based on individual preferences and daily schedules.

- *Benefits:* Provides flexibility and is less rigid than other methods. It allows individuals to adapt to fasting based on their lifestyle.

Spontaneous meal skipping refers to the unplanned decision to skip a meal, often due to factors such as lack of appetite, time constraints, or personal preference. While it may not follow a structured intermittent fasting schedule, spontaneous meal skipping shares some similarities with intermittent fasting approaches that involve periods of not eating. Here, we'll explore the potential effects, benefits, and considerations associated with spontaneous meal skipping.

Factors Influencing Spontaneous Meal Skipping.

- *Lack of Appetite:*

Sometimes, individuals may experience a lack of hunger or appetite, leading them to naturally skip a meal.

- *Busy Lifestyle:*

Time constraints or a hectic schedule can contribute to skipping meals, especially when individuals find it challenging to allocate time for regular eating.

- *Personal Preferences:*

Some individuals may practice spontaneous meal skipping based on personal preferences or intuitive eating, choosing to eat only when hungry.

- *Listen to Body Signals:*

Spontaneous meal skipping often involves paying attention to natural hunger and fullness cues, allowing individuals to eat in response to their body's signals.

Potential Benefits of Spontaneous Meal Skipping.

- *Caloric Reduction:*

Skipping a meal can naturally lead to a reduction in overall caloric intake, which may contribute to weight management.

- *Metabolic Flexibility:*

Intermittent periods of not eating, even if spontaneous, may enhance metabolic flexibility, encouraging the body to switch between burning glucose and fat for energy.

- *Insulin Sensitivity:*

Some studies suggest that occasional meal skipping may improve insulin sensitivity, supporting better blood sugar control.

- *Enhanced Focus and Productivity:*

Skipping a meal may lead to increased mental clarity for some individuals, potentially enhancing focus and productivity.

Considerations

- *Nutrient Intake:*

While spontaneous meal skipping can offer benefits, it's crucial to ensure that the overall diet remains balanced and provides essential nutrients when meals are consumed.

- *Individual Variation:*

Responses to spontaneous meal skipping can vary among individuals. Some people may feel energized and focused, while others may experience fatigue or irritability.

- *Hydration:* Staying well-hydrated is essential, especially when skipping meals. Water consumption is encouraged to maintain proper hydration levels.

- *Avoiding Compensatory Eating:*

After skipping a meal, individuals should avoid
compensating by overeating during subsequent
meals, as this can offset the potential benefits of
caloric reduction.

- *Consultation with Professionals:*
Individuals with existing health conditions, pregnant
or breastfeeding women, and those with specific
dietary requirements should consult with healthcare
or nutrition professionals before incorporating
spontaneous meal skipping into their routine.

Spontaneous meal skipping, when done intuitively
and without compensatory overeating, may offer
some potential benefits such as caloric reduction
and improved metabolic flexibility. However,
individual responses can vary, and it's essential to
approach spontaneous meal skipping with
awareness, considering overall nutritional needs and
consulting with professionals when necessary. As
with any dietary practice, moderation and balance
are key for long-term well-being.

❖ Circadian Fasting

- *Methodology:* Aligns fasting periods with the body's natural circadian rhythms. This often means fasting during the evening and overnight hours.

- *Benefits:* Supports the body's natural metabolic processes, potentially improving overall health. It may be more sustainable for those who find it challenging to fast during the day.

Circadian fasting is an approach to intermittent fasting that takes into account the body's natural circadian rhythms. This method aligns eating patterns with the body's internal clock, emphasizing the timing of meals in relation to the daily cycle of light and darkness. The core idea is that our metabolism and various physiological processes are influenced by the circadian rhythm, and syncing eating habits with this rhythm may optimize health and well-being.

Key Principles of Circadian Fasting

- *Time-Restricted Eating:*

Circadian fasting often involves time-restricted eating, where individuals limit their daily food intake to a specific time window. Commonly, this window is during daylight hours, aligning with the body's natural wakefulness and metabolic activity.

- *Morning Emphasis:*

Some proponents of circadian fasting recommend placing a higher emphasis on consuming larger meals earlier in the day. This aligns with the body's natural tendency for increased insulin sensitivity and metabolic activity during the morning.

- *Light Exposure:*

Exposure to natural light, especially in the morning, is considered important for regulating the circadian rhythm. This exposure may influence hunger and satiety signals, helping to synchronize the body's internal clock.

- *Avoiding Late-Night Eating:*

Circadian fasting often discourages late-night eating, as the body's metabolism tends to slow down in the evening. Consuming large meals close to bedtime may interfere with sleep quality and disrupt circadian rhythms.

Potential Benefits of Circadian Fasting

- *Improved Metabolic Health:*

Aligning eating patterns with circadian rhythms may enhance metabolic function, including improved insulin sensitivity and better blood sugar control.

- *Weight Management:*

Circadian fasting may contribute to weight management by optimizing the timing of nutrient intake, potentially influencing fat metabolism and energy balance.

- *Enhanced Sleep Quality:*

Avoiding late-night meals can positively impact sleep quality, as the digestive process is less active during the body's natural rest phase.

- *Hormonal Regulation:*

Circadian fasting may influence the secretion of hormones such as melatonin, cortisol, and growth hormone, which play key roles in regulating sleep, stress response, and metabolism.

Considerations

- *Individual Variability:*

The effectiveness of circadian fasting can vary among individuals. Factors such as lifestyle, work schedules, and personal preferences should be taken into account.

- *Nutrient-Dense Meals:*

While emphasizing timing, it's crucial to focus on nutrient-dense, balanced meals to meet nutritional needs and support overall health.

- *Hydration:*

Staying well-hydrated is important, and water consumption is typically encouraged during fasting periods.

- *Professional Guidance:*

Individuals with specific health conditions or those on medications should consult healthcare professionals or registered dietitians before adopting circadian fasting.

Circadian fasting is an approach to intermittent fasting that considers the body's natural circadian rhythms. By aligning eating patterns with the daily cycle of light and darkness, this method aims to optimize metabolic health, weight management, and overall well-being. As with any dietary approach, individualization, awareness, and professional guidance are essential for long-term success.

❖ Extended Fasting (24 hours or more)

- *Methodology:* Involves fasting for more extended periods, typically 24 hours or more. Extended fasts might be done occasionally or as part of a more extended fasting routine.
- *Benefits:* Allows for deeper autophagy and cellular repair. However, extended fasting requires careful planning and monitoring of nutrient intake.

Extended fasting, typically defined as abstaining from food for 24 hours or more, is a form of intermittent fasting that has gained attention for its potential health benefits. This approach involves more prolonged periods of not eating compared to shorter intermittent fasting methods. Extended fasting can vary in duration, ranging from 24 hours to several days, and it has been explored for its effects on metabolic health, cellular repair processes, and overall well-being.

Key Principles of Extended Fasting

- *Duration:*

Extended fasting usually involves fasting for a period exceeding 24 hours, often extending to 48 hours, 72 hours, or even longer.

- *Water and Hydration:*

While abstaining from food, individuals are encouraged to stay well-hydrated by consuming water, herbal teas, and electrolytes to maintain hydration and support bodily functions.

- *Periodic Fasting Cycles:*

Extended fasting is often practiced periodically, with individuals choosing to incorporate it into their routine at intervals ranging from weekly to monthly.

- *Nutrient-Dense Meals Pre and Post-Fast:* Prior to an extended fast, individuals may consume nutrient-dense meals to ensure the body is adequately nourished. Similarly, breaking the fast with balanced, nutritious foods is essential for a gradual reintroduction of nutrients.

Potential Benefits of Extended Fasting

- *Autophagy:* Extended fasting is associated with the induction of autophagy, a cellular process that involves the removal of damaged cells and cellular components. This process contributes to cellular repair and maintenance.

- *Insulin Sensitivity:* Some studies suggest that extended fasting may improve insulin sensitivity, potentially reducing the risk of insulin resistance and type 2 diabetes.

- **Fat Utilization:**

Extended fasting encourages the body to utilize stored fat for energy, which may contribute to weight loss and improvements in body composition.

- **Hormonal Regulation:**

Extended fasting can influence the secretion of hormones such as growth hormone, norepinephrine, and cortisol, which play roles in metabolism, stress response, and muscle preservation.

- **Mental Clarity:**

Some individuals report increased mental clarity and improved focus during extended fasting periods.

Considerations

- *Individual Tolerance:*

Extended fasting may not be suitable for everyone, and individual responses can vary. Some people may adapt well to longer fasting periods, while others may experience discomfort or adverse effects.

- *Hydration and Electrolytes:*

Maintaining proper hydration is crucial during extended fasting. Electrolyte supplementation may be necessary, especially during longer fasts.

- *Medical Monitoring:*

Individuals with existing health conditions, pregnant or breastfeeding women, and those on medications should consult healthcare professionals before attempting extended fasting.

- *Breaking the Fast Gradually:*

Breaking an extended fast should be done gradually with easily digestible, nutrient-dense foods to avoid digestive discomfort.

Extended fasting is an intermittent fasting approach that involves periods of abstaining from food for 24 hours or more. While it shows potential benefits for cellular repair, metabolic health, and weight management, it should be approached with caution, and individuals should consider their own health status and seek professional guidance when needed. As with any dietary approach, moderation, balance, and individualization are key factors for long-term success.

Understanding these different intermittent fasting methods enables individuals to choose an approach that aligns with their preferences, lifestyle, and health goals. Experimentation and flexibility are key to finding the most sustainable and effective fasting routine for each individual. Always consult with healthcare professionals before starting any significant dietary changes, especially if there are pre-existing health conditions.

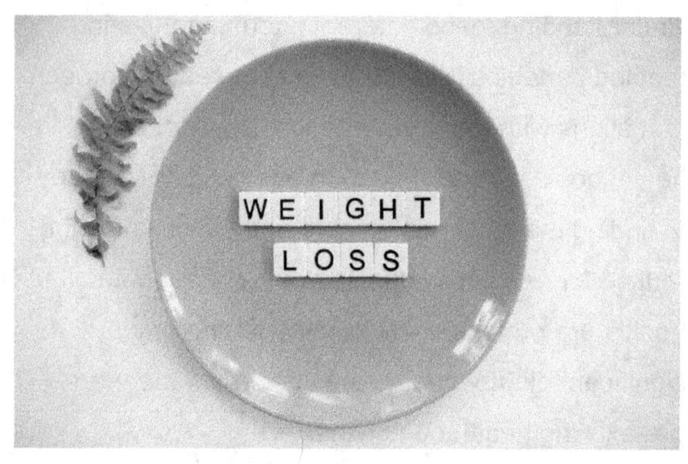

WEIGHT
LOSS

CHAPTER FOUR

Getting Started with Intermittent Fasting

Navigating Challenges

❖ Dealing With Hunger And Cravings

Understanding Hunger and Cravings:

- *Hunger:*

Recognize the difference between true physiological hunger and emotional or habitual triggers. True hunger is the body's signal for nourishment, while other cues might be linked to emotions, boredom, or routine.

- *Cravings:*

Cravings often involve a specific desire for a certain type of food. Identifying the triggers behind cravings can help manage them effectively.

Navigating hunger and cravings is a crucial aspect of successfully implementing Intermittent Fasting (IF). Here, we'll explore strategies and considerations for managing these sensations during different phases of an intermittent fasting routine.

- *Gradual Adjustment:*

Start by gradually increasing the fasting window. Begin with shorter fasting periods, such as 12-14 hours, and then gradually extend it over time. This allows your body to adapt to the new eating pattern, reducing hunger pangs.

- *Stay Hydrated:*

Drinking an adequate amount of water throughout the day can help curb hunger. Water not only keeps you hydrated but also makes you feel fuller, reducing the intensity of hunger.

- Opt for Protein and Healthy Fats:

Including protein-rich foods like lean meats, poultry, fish, eggs, and plant-based protein sources in your meals can help promote satiety. Additionally, incorporating healthy fats from sources like avocados, nuts, and olive oil can also help you feel fuller for longer.

- *Plan Balanced Meals:*

Ensure that your meals during the eating window are well-balanced, consisting of a variety of nutrients. A balanced meal with adequate protein, healthy fats, and carbohydrates can help keep hunger at bay.

- *Strategic Meal Timing:*

- Adjust Eating Window: If hunger or cravings are intense, consider adjusting your eating window. Experiment with different timings to find what suits your body's natural rhythms and preferences.

- *Include Fiber and Protein:*

- Fiber-Rich Foods: Fiber-rich foods, such as fruits, vegetables, and whole grains, can promote a feeling of fullness and help manage hunger.

- Protein: Including protein in your meals can also enhance satiety and prevent excessive hunger.

- *Mindful Eating:*

- Savor Meals: Make mindful eating a habit by appreciating every taste. This can help you connect with the sensory experience of eating and reduce the likelihood of overeating during your eating window.

- *Distract Yourself:*

- Engage in Activities: Engage in activities that divert your attention away from hunger or cravings. This could include going for a walk, reading a book, or participating in a hobby.

- *Progressive Fasting Approach:*

- Start Gradually: If you're new to intermittent fasting, consider starting with shorter fasting windows and gradually extending them as your body adapts.

- *Supplements and Herbs:*
- Consult a Professional: Consult healthcare professionals or a registered dietitian before using any supplements or herbs. Some may have appetite-suppressing effects, but their safety and efficacy vary.

- *Listen to Your Body:*
- Be Flexible:.Pay attention to how your body responds to intermittent fasting. If you're consistently experiencing severe hunger or cravings, it might be worth adjusting your approach or consulting with a healthcare professional.

- *Be Patient*:
- Adaptation Takes Time: Allow your body time to adapt to intermittent fasting. It's normal for hunger and cravings to fluctuate as your body adjusts to a new eating pattern.

Effectively navigating hunger and cravings during intermittent fasting involves a combination of mindful eating, balanced nutrition, hydration, and paying attention to your body's signals. Experiment with different strategies, be patient with the adaptation process, and prioritize your overall well-being. If challenges persist, consider seeking guidance from healthcare professionals or a registered dietitian to tailor an intermittent fasting plan that suits your individual needs and goals.

❖ Social Situations

- *- Challenge:*

Coordinating fasting schedules with social events.

- *- Navigation:*

Communicate your fasting routine to friends and family. Choose eating windows that align with social gatherings, and be flexible on occasion. The focus should be on socializing rather than solely on food..

Navigating social situations while practicing Intermittent Fasting (IF) can present unique challenges, especially since many social gatherings often revolve around meals. Here are strategies to help you manage social situations effectively while adhering to your intermittent fasting routine:

- *Communication:*

- Inform Others: Let friends and family know about your intermittent fasting plan. Explain that you have specific eating windows, so they understand your approach and can offer support.

- *Flexible Eating Windows:*

- Adjust Timing: Be flexible with your eating window if possible. If you have a social event that falls outside your usual eating window, consider adjusting it for that day to accommodate the situation.

- *Choose Wisely:*

- Smart Food Choices: When dining out or attending social events, make mindful food choices. Opt for nutrient-dense options and control portion sizes within your eating window.

- *Plan Ahead:*

- Pre-plan Meals: If you know you'll be attending a social event, plan your meals accordingly. Have a satisfying meal before the event to help you resist unhealthy or excessive food choices.

- **Intermittent Fasting Variations:**
- Consider Options: Explore intermittent fasting variations that might better suit your social schedule. For example, you might choose a method that allows for more flexibility on weekends or during special occasions.

- **Stay Hydrated:**
- Drink Water: Stay hydrated during social situations by drinking water or other non-caloric beverages. This can help you feel more satisfied and reduce the temptation to snack outside your eating window.

- **Practice Mindful Eating:**
- Savor Each Bite: When you do eat during social events, practice mindful eating. Savor each bite, enjoy the company, and focus on the social aspect rather than solely on the food.

- **Educate Others:**

- Share Benefits: Educate others about the potential health benefits of intermittent fasting. This can foster understanding and support from friends and family.

- Bring Your Own Food:
  - BYO Snacks:If you're unsure about the food options at an event, consider bringing a small snack or dish that aligns with your dietary preferences.

- Prioritize Enjoyment:
  - Balance is Key:While it's important to stick to your intermittent fasting plan, don't let it overshadow the enjoyment of social events. Find a balance that works for you and allows you to participate fully.

- Be Confident:
  - Own Your Choices:Be confident in your choice to practice intermittent fasting. Remember that your dietary decisions are personal, and it's okay to prioritize your health and well-being.

- Stay Positive:

- Focus on the Experience:Instead of fixating on
the food, focus on the social experience. Engage in
conversations, participate in activities, and enjoy the
overall atmosphere.

- Build a Support System:
- Find Like-Minded Individuals: Connect with
others who practice intermittent fasting. Having a
support system can make it easier to navigate social
situations and share tips and strategies.

Successfully navigating social situations during
intermittent fasting involves a combination of
effective communication, flexibility, planning, and
mindful choices. Prioritize your health and well-being
while still enjoying social events. Find a balance that
works for you, and remember that intermittent
fasting is a personal choice. By adopting a positive
and flexible mindset, you can make intermittent
fasting a sustainable part of your lifestyle while
participating in social activities.

❖ Energy Levels:

- Challenge: Potential energy fluctuations, especially during the adjustment phase.

- Navigation:Ensure sufficient sleep and consider adjusting the timing of fasting or eating periods based on when you feel most energized. Include nutrient-dense foods in meals to support energy levels.

Managing energy levels is a key aspect of a successful experience with Intermittent Fasting (IF). As your eating pattern changes, you may notice fluctuations in energy throughout the fasting and feeding windows. Here are strategies to navigate energy levels during different phases of intermittent fasting:

- Understand Initial Adjustments:
- Adaptation Period: Recognize that your body may need time to adapt to a new intermittent fasting routine. During the initial adjustment phase, energy levels might vary.

- Stay Hydrated:

- Water Intake:Dehydration can contribute to feelings of fatigue. Ensure you stay well-hydrated during both fasting and feeding periods by drinking water, herbal teas, or other non-caloric beverages.

3. Electrolyte Balance:

   - Include Electrolytes: Maintain proper electrolyte balance, especially if you experience symptoms like headaches or fatigue. Consider including electrolyte-rich foods or supplements, especially during fasting periods.

4. Strategic Meal Timing:

   - Meal Timing:Plan your meals strategically to align with your natural energy peaks. Some people find that having their main meal during a period of higher energy can enhance overall well-being.

5. Balanced Nutrition:

   - Nutrient-Dense Foods: Choose nutrient-dense foods during your eating window to provide a steady supply of energy. Include a mix of carbohydrates, proteins, and healthy fats to support sustained energy levels.

6. Avoid Extreme Caloric Deficits:

   - Adequate Calories: Ensure you're consuming an adequate number of calories during your eating window. Extreme caloric deficits can lead to fatigue and other negative effects on energy levels.

7. Prioritize Sleep:

   - Quality Sleep: Adequate and quality sleep is crucial for energy levels. Prioritize a consistent sleep schedule and create a sleep-friendly environment to support overall well-being.

8. Caffeine Moderation:

   - Caffeine Intake: Moderate caffeine intake can provide a temporary energy boost. However, excessive caffeine consumption, especially close to bedtime, may interfere with sleep quality.

9. Exercise Timing:

   - Strategic Exercise: Consider timing your exercise during periods of higher energy. Some people prefer working out during their fasting period, while others find it more beneficial during the feeding window.

10. Adapt to Your Body's Rhythms:

   - Listen to Your Body: Pay attention to your body's
natural rhythms and energy cycles. Adjust your
fasting and eating windows based on when you
naturally feel more alert and energetic.

11. Include Fiber and Protein:

   - Balanced Meals: Fiber and protein-rich foods
contribute to a feeling of fullness and can help
stabilize blood sugar levels, preventing energy
crashes.

12. Manage Stress:

   - Stress Reduction: Chronic stress can impact
energy levels. Incorporate stress-reducing activities
such as meditation, deep breathing, or other
relaxation techniques into your routine.

13. Be Patient and Flexible:

   - Adaptation Takes Time: Be patient as your body
adapts to intermittent fasting. If you experience low
energy initially, give it time, and be open to adjusting
your approach based on how your body responds.

Conclusion:

Navigating energy levels during intermittent fasting involves a combination of strategic planning, balanced nutrition, adequate hydration, and lifestyle adjustments. Pay attention to your body's signals, prioritize sleep and stress management, and be open to adapting your intermittent fasting approach to better suit your individual energy needs. By incorporating these strategies, you can optimize your energy levels and make intermittent fasting a sustainable and positive part of your lifestyle.

❖ Dehydration:

- Challenge: Forgetting to stay adequately hydrated during fasting periods.
- Navigation: Set reminders to drink water regularly. Consider adding electrolytes to water if needed. Herbal teas and infused water can also add variety while keeping you hydrated.

Dehydration is a concern that individuals practicing Intermittent Fasting (IF) should be mindful of, especially during fasting periods. Proper hydration is crucial for overall health, and dehydration can lead to a range of issues, including fatigue, dizziness, and impaired cognitive function. Here are strategies to navigate dehydration during IF:

- **Understand Fluid Needs:**
- Individual Variation: Fluid needs vary among individuals based on factors like age, weight, activity level, and climate. Consider these factors when determining your hydration requirements during IF.

- **Water Intake:**
- Consistent Hydration: Drink water consistently throughout the day, both during fasting and feeding periods. Adequate water intake is vital for various bodily functions, including digestion, nutrient transport, and temperature regulation.

- **Electrolyte Balance:**
- Include Electrolytes: Intermittent fasting can lead to electrolyte imbalances, especially if you're not consuming food regularly. Include electrolyte-rich

foods or consider adding electrolyte supplements to maintain balance.

- Monitor Urine Color:
  - Check Hydration Levels: Monitor the color of your urine as a rough indicator of hydration status. Light, pale yellow urine typically indicates proper hydration, while dark yellow or amber may suggest dehydration.

- Herbal Teas and Infusions:
  - Non-Caloric Options: Herbal teas and infusions can contribute to hydration without breaking your fast. Choose non-caloric options to avoid disrupting the fasting state.

- Avoid Excessive Caffeine:
  - Limit Caffeine: While moderate caffeine intake is generally considered hydrating, excessive caffeine can have a diuretic effect, potentially increasing fluid loss. Monitor your caffeine intake, especially if you're prone to dehydration.

- Hydrating Foods:

- Choose Hydrating Foods: Incorporate hydrating foods into your meals, such as fruits and vegetables with high water content. Cucumbers, watermelon, and celery are examples of hydrating food options.

- Pre-Fasting Hydration:
- Hydrate Before Fasting: Ensure you're well-hydrated before entering a fasting period. Drink water leading up to the start of your fast to establish a good hydration baseline.

- Sip Water Throughout the Day:
- Continuous Sipping: Rather than consuming large amounts of water at once, sip water consistently throughout the day. This approach helps maintain steady hydration levels.

- Address Thirst Promptly:
- Respond to Thirst: Pay attention to your body's signals. If you feel thirsty, respond promptly by drinking water. Thirst is an early indicator of dehydration.

- Rehydrate After Fasting:

- Gradual Rehydration: After a fasting period, gradually rehydrate rather than consuming large amounts of water quickly. This approach helps prevent discomfort and supports optimal hydration.

- Adjust for Climate and Activity Level:
- Climate Considerations: Hot or humid climates and increased physical activity can elevate fluid requirements. Adjust your water intake based on environmental conditions and your level of physical exertion.

- Listen to Your Body:
- Individual Needs: Individual hydration needs can vary. Listen to your body, and if you experience symptoms of dehydration, such as dizziness or fatigue, prioritize hydration.

Navigating dehydration during Intermittent Fasting involves a proactive approach to water intake, electrolyte balance, and monitoring your body's signals. By incorporating these strategies, you can maintain proper hydration levels, support your overall health, and enhance your experience with intermittent fasting. Remember that individual needs vary, so it's essential to find a hydration routine that works for you. If you have specific health concerns or conditions, consult with healthcare professionals or a registered dietitian for personalized guidance.

❖ Nutrient Intake

- Challenge: Ensuring proper nutrient intake within eating windows.

- Navigation: Plan well-balanced meals that include a variety of food groups. Consider consulting a nutritionist to ensure you meet your nutritional needs. If necessary, incorporate supplements to address potential deficiencies.

Navigating nutrient intake is a crucial aspect of ensuring that you meet your nutritional needs while practicing Intermittent Fasting (IF). While IF doesn't prescribe specific dietary guidelines, it's essential to focus on nutrient-dense foods and maintain a well-balanced diet to support overall health. Here are strategies to navigate nutrient intake during different phases of intermittent fasting:

- Prioritize Nutrient-Dense Foods:
- Whole Foods:Emphasize whole, nutrient-dense foods that provide a broad spectrum of essential nutrients. Fruits, vegetables, whole grains and healthy fats are all included in this.

- Balanced Meals:
- Macronutrient Balance: Aim for a balance of macronutrients (carbohydrates, proteins, and fats) in each meal to support various physiological functions and energy needs.

- Micronutrient-Rich Choices:
- Vitamins and Minerals: Ensure your meals include a variety of colorful fruits and vegetables to provide a range of vitamins and minerals. Different plant-based foods offer unique nutritional profiles.

- Hydrate with Nutrient-Rich Beverages:
- Herbal Teas, Infusions: Choose non-caloric beverages like herbal teas and infusions during

fasting periods to stay hydrated without adding unnecessary calories.

- Strategic Timing of Nutrient Intake:
- Meal Timing: Distribute nutrient intake strategically during your eating window. Consider consuming a mix of macronutrients early in your eating period to support energy levels.

- Fiber-Rich Foods:
- Whole Grains, Legumes: Include fiber-rich foods like whole grains, legumes, and vegetables to promote digestive health and enhance feelings of fullness.

- Protein Adequacy:
- Lean Protein Sources: Ensure you're getting an adequate amount of protein, which is essential for muscle maintenance and repair. Include lean protein sources such as poultry, fish, legumes, and tofu.

- Healthy Fats:

- Omega-3 Fatty Acids: Incorporate sources of healthy fats, particularly those rich in omega-3 fatty acids like fatty fish, flaxseeds, and walnuts.

- **Multivitamin Supplements (if needed):**
- Consult with a Professional: Consider multivitamin supplements if you have difficulty meeting your nutrient needs through food alone. However, prior to beginning any supplementation, it is imperative that you speak with a healthcare provider.

- **Avoid Overly Processed Foods:**
- Minimize Processed Foods: Limit the intake of highly processed and refined foods, as they may lack essential nutrients and contribute to an imbalanced diet.

- **Experiment with Different Eating Windows:**
- Personalized Approach: Experiment with different eating windows to find what suits your lifestyle and allows you to consume a well-balanced diet. Some

individuals may prefer larger meals, while others may opt for multiple smaller meals.

- **Consult with a Registered Dietitian:**
- Individualized Guidance: If you have specific dietary concerns, health conditions, or goals, consider consulting with a registered dietitian. They can provide personalized guidance on meeting your nutritional needs with intermittent fasting.

- **Listen to Your Body:**
- Individual Responses: Pay attention to how your body responds to different foods and eating patterns. Everyone is unique, and your nutritional needs may vary based on factors like age, activity level, and health status.

Navigating nutrient intake during Intermittent Fasting involves a mindful and intentional approach to food choices. Prioritize nutrient-dense, whole foods, and aim for a well-balanced diet that supports your overall health and well-being. Tailor your nutritional strategy based on your individual preferences, lifestyle, and health goals. If you have specific dietary concerns or health conditions, seek guidance from healthcare professionals or a registered dietitian for personalized advice.

❖ Exercise Timing:

- Challenge: Finding the right time to exercise during fasting periods.

- Navigation: Experiment with different exercise timings to see what works for you. Some individuals prefer working out during fasting, while others find it more comfortable during eating windows. Listen to your body's signals.

Navigating exercise timing is a key consideration for individuals practicing Intermittent Fasting (IF). Properly timed physical activity can complement the effects of intermittent fasting and contribute to overall health and fitness. Here are strategies to navigate exercise timing during different phases of intermittent fasting:

- Understand Individual Preferences:

- Personal Rhythms: Consider your individual preferences and rhythms when it comes to physical activity. Some people may prefer exercising in a fasted state, while others may find it more comfortable after eating.

- Morning Workouts:
- Benefits: Exercising in the morning, especially during the fasting period, may enhance fat utilization for energy and potentially support weight management. Additionally, it can contribute to increased alertness and improved mood throughout the day.

- Evening Workouts:
- Benefits: Evening workouts, particularly during the feeding window, allow you to replenish glycogen stores after exercise and provide essential nutrients for muscle recovery. This timing might be suitable for those who prefer a larger meal post-workout.

- Cardiovascular Exercise in Fasted State:
- Cardio Benefits: Performing cardiovascular exercises in a fasted state may encourage the body

to use stored fat for energy, potentially aiding in fat loss. Individual reactions do differ, though, so pay attention to your body.

- **Strength Training in Fed State:**
- Muscle Preservation: Strength training during the feeding window allows for adequate protein intake, which is crucial for muscle preservation, repair, and growth.

- **Hydration:**
- Pre-Exercise Hydration: Regardless of when you choose to exercise, ensure you're adequately hydrated before starting your workout. Performance and recuperation can be severely impacted by dehydration.

- **Post-Workout Nutrition:**
- Refuel Appropriately: After exercising, pay attention to post-workout nutrition. Consume a balanced meal or snack with both carbohydrates and protein to replenish glycogen stores and support muscle recovery.

- Experiment with Timing:

- Find Your Optimal Time: Experiment with different exercise timings to discover what feels best for you. It may take some trial and error to determine whether fasted or fed workouts suit your energy levels and preferences.

- Listen to Your Body:

- Individual Responses: Pay attention to how your body responds to exercise at different times. Some people may feel more energized and perform better in a fasted state, while others may prefer exercising after a meal.

- Consider Type of Exercise:

- Activity-Specific Timing: The type of exercise can influence optimal timing. High-intensity workouts might be better suited for the fed state, while low to moderate-intensity activities may be comfortable during fasting.

- Professional Guidance:

- Consult with Experts: If you have specific fitness goals or health concerns, consider consulting with fitness professionals or healthcare providers. They can offer guidance on how to align your exercise routine with intermittent fasting.

- Gradual Adaptation:
  - Allow Time for Adaptation: If you're new to exercising during intermittent fasting, allow your body time to adapt. Gradually incorporate physical activity and monitor how it affects your energy levels and overall well-being.

- Balance with Recovery:
  - Prioritize Recovery: Balance your exercise routine with adequate recovery time. Rest and proper sleep are essential components of overall health and fitness.

Navigating exercise timing during Intermittent Fasting involves finding a balance that aligns with your preferences, energy levels, and fitness goals. Whether you choose to exercise in a fasted or fed state, prioritizing hydration, proper nutrition, and recovery are crucial. Listen to your body, be open to experimentation, and consider seeking guidance from fitness professionals or healthcare providers to tailor your exercise routine to your individual needs.

❖ Overeating during Eating Windows:

- Challenge: Temptation to overeat when breaking the fast.

- Navigation: Start with a small, balanced meal to prevent excessive calorie consumption. To satisfy your nutritional needs, put your attention on nutrient-dense foods. Practice mindful eating to recognize satiety cues.

Navigating overeating during eating windows is a common concern for individuals practicing Intermittent Fasting (IF). While IF can be an effective tool for weight management, it's essential to approach eating windows mindfully to avoid overconsumption. Here are strategies to navigate overeating during different phases of intermittent fasting:

- **Mindful Eating:**
- Present Awareness: Practice mindful eating by being fully present during meals. Take note of each bite's flavor, texture, and level of satisfaction. This can help prevent mindless overeating.

- **Slow and Enjoyable Meals:**
- Chew Carefully: Give each bite your full attention. Eating slowly allows your body to recognize signals of fullness, reducing the likelihood of overeating.

- **Balanced Macronutrients:**
- Protein, Fats, Carbs: Include a balance of macronutrients in your meals. Protein, healthy fats, and complex carbohydrates contribute to satiety and help prevent excessive eating.

- **Proper Hydration:**
- Drink Water Before Meals: Drink water before meals to help you feel more full and satisfied. Hunger pangs can occasionally be indicators of dehydration.

- **Planned Meals:**

- Meal Preparation: Plan your meals in advance and have them prepared. Knowing what you will eat can reduce the chances of impulsive overeating or reaching for unhealthy options.

- Avoiding Extreme Hunger:
- Regular Meals: Aim for regular, balanced meals to avoid extreme hunger during eating windows. Extreme hunger can lead to rapid, uncontrolled eating.

- Control Portions:
- Use Smaller Plates: Opt for smaller plates to control portion sizes. This visual trick can help you feel satisfied with smaller amounts of food.

- Pay attention to your body's signals of hunger and fullness. Stop eating when you feel satisfied rather than waiting until you're overly full.

- Avoiding Emotional Eating:
- Address Emotional Triggers: Be mindful of emotional eating triggers. If you often find yourself

reaching for food to soothe yourself or decompress, consider other coping strategies like working out, practicing meditation, or speaking with a friend.

- Quality Over Quantity:
- Choose Nutrient-Dense Foods: Prioritize nutrient-dense foods over calorie-dense options. Quality matters, and choosing nutrient-rich foods can help meet your nutritional needs without overeating.

- Reevaluate Food Choices:
- Reflect on Food Choices: Periodically evaluate the nutritional value of your food choices. If you notice patterns of overeating certain types of foods, reassess your choices for better balance.

- Social Eating Awareness:
- Mindful Social Eating: When dining with others, stay mindful of your own hunger and fullness cues. Social situations can sometimes lead to overeating due to external cues.

- Regular Physical Activity:

- Exercise Routine: Incorporate regular physical activity into your routine. Exercise can support weight management and enhance overall well-being.

- Professional Guidance:
- Consult with Professionals: If you struggle with overeating, consider seeking guidance from healthcare professionals or registered dietitians. They can provide personalized advice to address your specific challenges.

- Learn from Experiences:
- Reflect on Patterns: Reflect on instances of overeating and learn from them. Understand the factors contributing to overconsumption and implement strategies to address those factors in the future.

Navigating overeating during eating windows in Intermittent Fasting involves adopting mindful eating practices, controlling portions, and making intentional food choices. By staying present during meals, prioritizing nutrient-dense foods, and addressing emotional triggers, you can create a healthier relationship with food within the context of intermittent fasting. If overeating persists as a concern, seeking guidance from healthcare professionals or registered dietitians can provide valuable support and personalized strategies.

❖ Digestive Issues:

 - Challenge: Some may experience digestive discomfort during fasting or when reintroducing food.
 - Navigation: Gradually introduce fasting periods and adjust eating patterns based on digestive responses. Include fiber-rich foods to support digestive health

Navigating digestive issues during Intermittent Fasting (IF) involves understanding how fasting periods and meal timing can affect the digestive system. While some individuals may experience improved digestion with IF, others might encounter challenges. Here are strategies to navigate digestive issues during different phases of intermittent fasting:

- Gradual Adaptation:

 - Allow Time for Adjustment: If you're new to intermittent fasting, give your digestive system time to adapt. Sudden changes in eating patterns may initially cause discomfort, but gradual adaptation can help alleviate digestive issues.

- Hydration:

 - Drink Plenty of Water: Stay well-hydrated during fasting and eating windows. Water supports digestion and helps prevent issues like constipation. Dehydration can exacerbate digestive discomfort.

- Choose Fiber-Rich Foods:

 - Include Fiber in Meals: Consume fiber-rich foods like fruits, vegetables, whole grains, and legumes. Fiber promotes healthy digestion by adding bulk to stool and supporting regular bowel movements.

- Probiotic-Rich Foods:

 - Incorporate Probiotics: Include probiotic-rich foods like yogurt, kefir, sauerkraut, and kimchi. Probiotics support gut health by promoting the growth of beneficial bacteria.

- **Meal Timing Considerations:**
- Evaluate Meal Timing: Assess whether the timing of your meals during the eating window affects your digestion. Some individuals may experience better digestion with specific meal timings.

- **Avoid Overeating:**
- Control Portion Sizes: Overeating can strain the digestive system. Control portion sizes and listen to your body's signals of fullness to prevent digestive discomfort.

- **Mindful Eating Practices:**
- Chew Thoroughly: Practice mindful eating by chewing your food thoroughly. Proper chewing aids in the digestion process and reduces the risk of indigestion.

- **Avoid Highly Processed Foods:**
- Minimize Processed Foods: Limit the intake of highly processed and refined foods, as they may

contribute to digestive issues. Opt for whole, minimally processed options.

● Limit Caffeine and Spicy Foods:
- Moderate Stimulants: Excessive caffeine and spicy foods can irritate the digestive tract. Moderate your intake to assess their impact on your digestive comfort.

Navigating digestive issues during Intermittent Fasting involves a combination of mindful eating, hydration, and adjustments to fasting and eating patterns. Listening to your body, staying hydrated, and incorporating gut-friendly foods can contribute to improved digestive comfort. If issues persist, seeking guidance from healthcare professionals can help identify underlying causes and provide tailored solutions for a more comfortable experience with intermittent fasting.

❖ Long-Term Sustainability:

- Challenge: Maintaining IF as a sustainable lifestyle.

- Navigation: Emphasize flexibility and find a fasting routine that aligns with your preferences and daily life. Periodically reassess and adjust your approach to ensure it remains realistic and enjoyable.

Navigating long-term sustainability with Intermittent Fasting (IF) involves adopting a balanced and flexible approach that aligns with your lifestyle, preferences, and health goals. Sustainable practices ensure that IF becomes a lasting and positive aspect of your routine. Here are key strategies to promote long-term sustainability with intermittent fasting:

- **Personalized Approach:**
  - Tailor to Your Preferences: Customize your intermittent fasting plan to suit your preferences. Whether it's a specific fasting method, meal timing, or duration of fasting periods, adapt IF to align with your lifestyle.

- **Gradual Implementation:**

- Start Slowly: If you're new to IF, start with a gradual approach. Begin with shorter fasting windows and progressively extend them as your body adapts. This can enhance the sustainability of the practice.

- Consistency Over Rigidity:
- Flexible Schedule: Aim for consistency but be flexible with your IF schedule. Life can be unpredictable, and allowing for adaptability promotes sustainability. Adjust fasting periods based on social events, work commitments, or personal preferences.

- Nutrient-Dense Eating:
- Prioritize Nutrition: Focus on nutrient-dense foods during your eating windows. Emphasize a balanced intake of proteins, healthy fats, fruits, vegetables, and whole grains to support overall health.

- Hydration:
- Stay Hydrated: Proper hydration is essential for overall well-being. Drink water, herbal teas, and

other non-caloric beverages throughout the day to support hydration during fasting periods.

- Regular Exercise:
- Incorporate Physical Activity: Integrate regular physical activity into your routine. Exercise not only complements IF but also contributes to overall health and well-being.

- Listen to Your Body:
- Individualized Approach: Pay attention to your body's signals. If you're feeling fatigued, excessively hungry, or experiencing discomfort, consider adjusting your fasting approach. Listen to what works best for you.

- Social Adaptation:
- Navigate Social Situations: Develop strategies to handle social situations while practicing IF. Communicate your eating schedule to friends and family, or adjust your fasting windows to accommodate social events.

- Regular Health Check-ups:

- Monitor Health: Schedule regular check-ups with healthcare professionals to monitor your overall health. IF should be a complement to a healthy lifestyle, and it's important to ensure it aligns with your individual needs.

- **Address Emotional Aspects:**
- Mindful Eating Practices: Address emotional aspects of eating by incorporating mindful eating practices. Be aware of emotional triggers and cultivate a positive relationship with food.

- **Educate Yourself:**
- Continuous Learning: Stay informed about the science and principles behind IF. Understanding the physiological effects can enhance your commitment and confidence in the long-term sustainability of the practice.

- **Regular Review and Adaptation:**
- Assess Progress: Periodically assess your progress and how IF fits into your life. Be open to adjusting your approach based on changes in your goals, lifestyle, or health requirements.

- Community and Support:

- Connect with Others: Join communities or seek support from individuals practicing IF. Sharing experiences, tips, and challenges with like-minded individuals can provide encouragement and motivation.

- Maintain a Balanced Lifestyle:

- Holistic Approach: Embrace a holistic approach to health. Intermittent fasting is one element of a healthy lifestyle that includes proper nutrition, physical activity, stress management, and sufficient sleep.

- Professional Guidance:

- Consult with Experts: If you have specific health concerns or conditions, consult with healthcare professionals or a registered dietitian. They can provide personalized guidance and ensure that IF aligns with your individual health needs.

Long-term sustainability with Intermittent Fasting requires a balanced, flexible, and individualized approach. By customizing IF to fit your lifestyle, prioritizing nutritional quality, and staying attuned to your body's signals, you can foster a sustainable and positive relationship with this eating pattern. Regular evaluation, adaptation, and seeking professional guidance contribute to a lasting and beneficial experience with intermittent fasting.

❖ Consulting Professionals:

- Challenge: Addressing health concerns or uncertainties about IF.

- Navigation: Consult healthcare professionals or a registered dietitian before starting intermittent fasting, especially if you have underlying health conditions. They can provide personalized guidance and monitor your progress.

Consulting with professionals, such as healthcare providers and registered dietitians, is a prudent and valuable step when considering or practicing Intermittent Fasting (IF). These professionals can offer personalized guidance based on your individual health status, goals, and any underlying medical conditions. Here's an in-depth exploration of the importance and considerations for consulting professionals during IF:

- Individual Health Assessment:
- Pre-existing Conditions: Healthcare professionals can conduct a thorough assessment of your health, taking into account any pre-existing medical conditions, medications, or individual health concerns. This ensures that IF aligns with your specific health needs.

- Personalized Guidance:
- Tailored Recommendations: Registered dietitians can provide personalized nutrition advice that considers your dietary preferences, lifestyle, and health goals. This tailored approach enhances the effectiveness and safety of IF.

- Risk Evaluation:
- Identifying Risks: Professionals can help identify potential risks associated with IF, especially for individuals with certain health conditions. This

includes monitoring for signs of nutrient deficiencies, electrolyte imbalances, or issues related to blood sugar regulation.

- Nutritional Adequacy:
- Ensuring Nutrient Intake: Dietitians can assess the nutritional adequacy of your IF plan to ensure you're meeting your daily nutrient requirements. This is crucial for sustaining overall health and preventing nutrient deficiencies.

- Weight Management Support:
- Holistic Approach: For those pursuing IF for weight management, professionals can offer a holistic approach that includes not only fasting strategies but also guidance on balanced nutrition, exercise, and behavior modification.

- Adaptation for Medical Conditions:
- Medical Conditions: Individuals with conditions such as diabetes, cardiovascular issues, or hormonal imbalances may benefit from professional guidance to adapt IF safely. Healthcare providers

can help tailor fasting approaches to manage specific health concerns.

- Medication Adjustments:

- Monitoring Medications: Healthcare professionals can monitor and adjust medications if necessary, as the timing and composition of meals during IF may influence the effectiveness or side effects of certain medications.

- Monitoring Blood Parameters:

- Regular Check-ups: Regular blood tests and health check-ups can help monitor changes in key parameters like blood glucose, lipid levels, and other metabolic markers. This allows for early detection of any issues related to IF.

- Behavioral Support:

- Addressing Habits: Dietitians can provide behavioral support to address eating habits, emotional triggers, and any psychological aspects related to food. This can contribute to a more positive and sustainable experience with IF.

- Managing Disordered Eating:

- Eating Disorders: For individuals with a history of or susceptibility to eating disorders, professionals can provide specialized support to prevent the development or exacerbation of disordered eating patterns.

- Pregnancy and Lactation:

- Special Considerations: Professionals can offer specific guidance for individuals who are pregnant or lactating, as nutritional needs are heightened during these periods. IF may need to be adapted to ensure adequate nutrient intake.

- Adjustments for Aging:

- Aging Considerations: Professionals can consider age-related factors when advising on IF. Older adults may have different nutritional needs and considerations, and a tailored approach can help address these.

- Monitoring Mental Health:

- Addressing Stress: Healthcare professionals can assess the impact of IF on mental health, especially regarding stress levels and emotional well-being. Strategies to manage stress can be incorporated into your overall health plan.

- Educational Support:
- Guidance and Information: Professionals can provide education on the science and principles behind IF, ensuring that individuals have accurate information and understand the physiological effects on the body.

- Regular Follow-ups:
- Monitoring Progress: Regular follow-ups with healthcare professionals or dietitians allow for ongoing monitoring of your health and progress with IF. Adjustments can be made based on your evolving needs and goals.

Consulting with professionals during Intermittent Fasting is a proactive and essential step to ensure the safety, effectiveness, and long-term sustainability of your dietary approach. Whether it's a healthcare provider for overall health assessment or a registered dietitian for personalized nutrition guidance, these professionals play a crucial role in tailoring IF to your individual needs and circumstances. Regular communication and collaboration with professionals contribute to a positive and health-focused experience with intermittent fasting.

Navigating challenges during intermittent fasting involves a combination of adaptation, flexibility, and mindful planning. By addressing specific concerns and adjusting your approach based on individual needs, intermittent fasting can become a sustainable and rewarding part of your lifestyle.

CHAPTER FIVE

Combining Intermittent Fasting (IF) with exercise

Combining Intermittent Fasting (IF) with exercise can be a synergistic approach to enhance overall health, improve fitness levels, and support weight management. However, it's essential to approach this combination mindfully to ensure that both fasting and exercise align with your individual needs and goals. Here's an extensive exploration of the benefits, considerations, and strategies for combining intermittent fasting with exercise:

Benefits of Combining IF with Exercise

* Enhanced Fat Utilization:

- Synergistic Fat Burning: Exercising in a fasted state may encourage the body to utilize stored fat for energy, potentially enhancing fat burning. Those who are trying to lose weight may find this helpful.

* Improved Insulin Sensitivity:

- Combined Metabolic Benefits: The combination of IF and exercise can improve insulin sensitivity. Regular physical activity complements fasting by aiding in glucose regulation and enhancing metabolic health.

* Muscle Preservation and Growth:

- Optimal Protein Utilization: Pairing IF with resistance training supports muscle preservation and growth. Consuming adequate protein during eating windows becomes crucial to support these muscle-related goals.

- Adaptation to Fasting:
- Training the Body: Exercise during fasting periods can help the body adapt to fasting conditions, making the overall fasting experience more manageable over time.

- Enhanced Autophagy:
- Cellular Cleanup: Both IF and exercise stimulate autophagy, a process that involves the removal of damaged cells and cellular components. This contributes to cellular health and longevity.

Considerations for Combining IF with Exercise

- Individual Variability:

- Listen to Your Body:Individual responses to combining IF with exercise can vary. Pay attention to how your body responds to different types, intensities, and timings of exercise during fasting periods.

- **Timing of Exercise:**
- Experiment with Timing: Experiment with the timing of your workouts to find what works best for you. Some individuals prefer fasted workouts in the morning, while others may opt for exercising during eating windows.

- **Nutrient Timing:**
- Post-Workout Nutrition: After exercising, prioritize post-workout nutrition to support recovery. Include a mix of protein and carbohydrates in your post-exercise meal to replenish glycogen stores and aid muscle repair.

- **Hydration:**
- Stay Hydrated: Hydration is crucial, especially when combining fasting and exercise. Drink water

regularly to maintain fluid balance and support overall performance.

- **Electrolyte Balance:**
  - Include Electrolytes: Intense or prolonged exercise during fasting periods may increase the need for electrolytes. Consider including electrolyte-rich foods or supplements to maintain balance.

- **Type of Exercise:**
  - Adapt to Fasting: High-intensity workouts might be more challenging during fasting periods, while low to moderate-intensity exercises may be more comfortable. Adjust the intensity based on your fasting state and energy levels.

- **Professional Guidance:**
  - Consult with Experts: If you have specific health concerns or are new to exercise and fasting, consult with healthcare professionals or fitness experts. They can provide guidance tailored to your individual needs and goals.

Strategies for Combining IF with Exercise

- Start Gradually:

- Adaptation Period: If you're new to both IF and exercise, start gradually. Allow your body time to adapt to fasting and incorporate exercise progressively.

- Diverse Workouts:

- Mix of Cardio and Strength: Include a variety of workouts, combining cardiovascular exercises with strength training. This ensures a well-rounded fitness routine.

- Meal Planning:

- Pre-Workout and Post-Workout Meals: Plan your meals to include pre-workout and post-workout nutrition. This helps optimize performance, recovery, and overall energy levels.

- Assess Energy Levels:

- Adapt to Energy Levels: Pay attention to your energy levels during fasting and adjust your exercise intensity accordingly. If you feel fatigued, consider lower-intensity workouts.

- **Rest and Recovery:**
- Prioritize Rest Days: Include rest days in your routine to allow for adequate recovery. Rest is crucial for preventing overtraining and promoting overall well-being.

- **Consult with a Dietitian:**
- Nutritional Guidance: Consult with a registered dietitian to ensure your dietary choices support both fasting and exercise. They can provide personalized nutritional guidance based on your goals.

- **Track Progress:**
- Monitor Fitness Gains: Keep track of your fitness progress, including strength gains, endurance improvements, and changes in body composition. Adjust your exercise routine as needed.

- **Regular Health Check-ups:**
- Overall Health Monitoring: Schedule regular check-ups with healthcare professionals to monitor

your overall health. This includes assessing cardiovascular health, bone density, and other factors relevant to both fasting and exercise.

Combining Intermittent Fasting with exercise can be a powerful approach for improving overall health and fitness. By paying attention to individual variability, adjusting exercise timing and intensity, and seeking professional guidance when needed, you can create a sustainable and effective routine that aligns with your goals. Regular assessment of your progress and adaptation to your body's signals contribute to a balanced and beneficial experience with both IF and exercise.

Optimal Workouts During Fasting

Choosing optimal workouts during fasting periods involves considering factors such as energy levels, workout intensity, and individual preferences. The type of exercise you select can impact how well your body performs in a fasted state. Here are some workout options that may be well-suited for fasting periods:

- Low to Moderate-Intensity Cardiovascular Exercise:

- Benefits: Walking, cycling, or jogging at a steady pace can be effective during fasting. These activities help burn calories, enhance cardiovascular health, and may be more comfortable in a fasted state compared to high-intensity workouts.

- Yoga and Pilates:

- Benefits: Yoga and Pilates focus on bodyweight movements, flexibility, and controlled breathing. These exercises are generally lower in intensity and can be suitable during fasting periods, promoting mindfulness and enhancing flexibility.

- Bodyweight Workouts:

- Benefits: Exercises like bodyweight squats, lunges, push-ups, and planks can be effective for strength training during fasting. They don't require equipment, and the intensity can be adjusted based on your fitness level.

- Circuit Training:

- Benefits: Circuits that combine both cardiovascular and resistance exercises can provide a comprehensive workout. Adjust the intensity based on your energy levels, and include short rest intervals between exercises.

- Swimming:
- Benefits: Swimming is a low-impact exercise that engages multiple muscle groups. The buoyancy of water reduces stress on joints, making it a suitable option during fasting periods.

- Hiking:
- Benefits: Hiking offers a combination of cardiovascular exercise and exposure to nature. It can be adapted to different fitness levels, making it an enjoyable option during fasting.

- Light Resistance Training:
- Benefits: Incorporating light resistance training with resistance bands or light dumbbells can be effective. Focus on higher repetitions and lower weights to maintain form and prevent excessive strain.

- Stretching and Mobility Exercises:

- Benefits: Stretching and mobility exercises can enhance flexibility and reduce muscle tension. They are gentle on the body and can be particularly beneficial during fasting for promoting overall well-being.

Considerations for Optimal Workouts During Fasting

- Listen to Your Body:

- Individual Responses: Pay attention to how your body responds to different types of exercise during fasting. Everyone reacts differently, so choose activities that feel comfortable for you.

- Hydration:

- Stay Hydrated: Ensure proper hydration, especially during workouts in a fasted state. Drink water before, during, and after your exercise session to prevent dehydration.

- Pre-Workout Nutrition:

- Consider a Balanced Snack: If you find that you need some energy before a workout, consider a small, balanced snack containing carbohydrates and protein. This may assist in maintaining your energy levels.

- **Post-Workout Nutrition:**
- Replenish with Nutrient-Dense Foods: After your workout, prioritize nutrient-dense foods that include both carbohydrates and protein to replenish glycogen stores and support muscle recovery.

- **Timing of Workouts:**
- Experiment with Timing: Explore different times of the day for your workouts during fasting periods. Some individuals may feel more energetic in the morning, while others prefer later in the day.

- **Adjust Intensity:**
- Modify Intensity Levels: If you're feeling fatigued during fasting, consider lowering the intensity of your workout. Focus on maintaining a steady pace and form to avoid excessive strain.

- Professional Guidance:

- Consult with Experts: If you have specific health concerns or are unsure about the most suitable workouts during fasting, consult with healthcare professionals or fitness experts for personalized advice.

Optimal workouts during fasting periods depend on individual preferences, fitness levels, and comfort. Low to moderate-intensity exercises, bodyweight workouts, and activities like yoga or swimming can be well-tailored for fasting. Always listen to your body, stay hydrated, and consider seeking professional guidance to create a workout routine that aligns with your goals and supports your overall well-being during intermittent fasting.

Maximizing Fitness Benefits

Maximizing fitness benefits involves a holistic approach that includes not only exercise but also considerations for nutrition, recovery, and overall lifestyle. Whether you're practicing Intermittent

Fasting (IF) or following a regular eating pattern, here are key strategies to optimize fitness gains:

- Balanced Nutrition:
- Prioritize Nutrient-Dense Foods: Focus on a balanced diet that includes a variety of nutrient-dense foods. Ensure an adequate intake of proteins, healthy fats, carbohydrates, vitamins, and minerals to support overall health and fitness.

- Protein Intake:
- Adequate Protein: Consume sufficient protein to support muscle repair, growth, and maintenance. Protein-rich foods such as lean meats, fish, dairy, legumes, and plant-based sources can contribute to optimal fitness outcomes.

- Hydration:
- Optimal Fluid Intake: Stay well-hydrated, as water is essential for various physiological processes, including nutrient transport, temperature regulation, and joint lubrication. Hydration is crucial for overall fitness and performance.

- **Pre-Workout Nutrition:**

- Balanced Snack: If exercising in a fasted state, consider a balanced snack with both carbohydrates and protein before the workout to provide energy and support performance.

- **Post-Workout Nutrition:**

- Recovery Nutrition: Consume a post-workout meal or snack containing protein and carbohydrates to replenish glycogen stores and support muscle recovery. This is crucial for maximizing the benefits of your exercise routine.

- **Diverse Workouts:**

- Mix of Exercises: Include a variety of exercises in your routine, encompassing cardiovascular, strength training, flexibility, and balance exercises. Diverse workouts contribute to overall fitness and prevent plateaus.

- **Consistent Exercise Routine:**

- Regular Physical Activity: Establish a consistent exercise routine. Regularity is key for long-term fitness gains. Aim for a balance between cardiorespiratory exercise, strength training, and flexibility exercises.

- Progressive Overload:
  - Gradual Intensity Increase: Incorporate progressive overload by gradually increasing the intensity, duration, or resistance of your workouts. This helps challenge your body and promotes continual improvement.

- Rest and Recovery:
  - Adequate Rest: Allow time for rest and recovery. Muscles need time to repair and adapt to exercise stress. Ensure sufficient sleep, incorporate rest days, and practice relaxation techniques to support recovery.

- Quality Sleep:
  - - Make Sleep a Priority: Getting a good night's sleep is crucial to general health and fitness. Try to get between seven and nine hours of sleep every night. Sleep influences recovery, cognitive function, and hormonal balance.

- **Stress Management:**
- Mind-Body Practices: Incorporate stress-management techniques such as meditation, deep breathing, or yoga. Chronic stress can negatively impact fitness gains, so fostering a balanced lifestyle is crucial.

- **Professional Guidance:**
- Consult with Experts: If you have specific fitness goals or health concerns, consider seeking guidance from fitness professionals or healthcare providers. They can provide personalized advice and support your fitness journey.

- **Periodic Assessments:**
- Evaluate Progress: Periodically assess your fitness progress. Track changes in strength, endurance, flexibility, and overall well-being. Adjust your routine based on your evolving goals and capabilities.

- **Consistency Over Intensity:**
- Steady Commitment: Consistency in your fitness routine is more crucial than occasional intense

workouts. Sustainable, long-term commitment yields better results and reduces the risk of burnout or injury.

- Enjoyment Factor:
- Choose Enjoyable Activities: Engage in activities you enjoy. Whether it's dancing, hiking, cycling, or weightlifting, the enjoyment factor increases adherence to your fitness routine, making it more sustainable.

Maximizing fitness benefits involves a comprehensive approach that integrates nutrition, exercise, recovery, and overall well-being. By prioritizing balanced nutrition, diverse workouts, proper hydration, and incorporating rest and recovery strategies, you can optimize the outcomes of your fitness efforts. Consistency, progressive overload, and enjoyment contribute to a sustainable and fulfilling fitness journey.

Intermittent Fasting and Health Conditions

Intermittent Fasting (IF) can impact health conditions in various ways, and its effects may vary depending on individual health status. Here's a brief overview of the relationship between intermittent fasting and certain health conditions:

- Type 2 Diabetes:

- Positive Impact: IF may improve insulin sensitivity and help regulate blood sugar levels. However, individuals with diabetes should consult healthcare professionals before starting IF to ensure a safe and personalized approach.

- Cardiovascular Health:

- Potential Benefits: IF might have positive effects on cardiovascular health, including improved lipid profiles and blood pressure. Nevertheless, those with existing heart conditions should seek guidance from healthcare providers.

- Obesity:
- Weight Management: IF is often used for weight management, as it may help reduce calorie intake and promote fat loss. Consultation with healthcare professionals is advisable, especially for those with obesity-related health issues.

- Neurological Disorders:
- Research in Progress: Some studies suggest that IF could have neuroprotective effects, potentially benefiting conditions like Alzheimer's or Parkinson's. Nevertheless, additional investigation is required to establish definitive proof.

- Hormonal Conditions:
- Caution Advised: Individuals with hormonal imbalances, such as thyroid disorders or polycystic ovary syndrome (PCOS), should approach IF cautiously and under the guidance of healthcare professionals.

- Gastrointestinal Issues:

- Mixed Effects: IF may influence gut health positively for some, but others may experience digestive issues. Individuals with pre-existing gastrointestinal conditions should consult with healthcare providers.

- **Pregnancy and Lactation:**
- Not Recommended: IF is generally not recommended during pregnancy and lactation. Adequate nutrition is crucial during these periods, and any dietary changes should be discussed with healthcare providers.

- **Eating Disorders:**
- Caution Advised: IF may pose challenges for individuals with a history of or susceptibility to eating disorders. It's essential to prioritize mental and emotional well-being and consult with healthcare professionals for personalized advice.

- **Chronic Illness:**
- Individual Considerations: Individuals with chronic illnesses should approach IF with caution and seek guidance from healthcare providers. The

impact of fasting can vary based on the specific health condition.

- **Medication Interaction:**
- Adjustments may be Needed: Some medications may need adjustments in timing or dosage during fasting. Individuals on medications should consult with healthcare professionals to ensure proper management.

- **Overall Health Assessment:**
- Consult Healthcare Professionals: Before starting IF, it's advisable for individuals with health conditions to undergo a comprehensive health assessment. Health care providers are able to offer tailored guidance according to each patient's unique condition.

Conclusion:

While intermittent fasting may offer potential health benefits, its suitability for individuals with specific health conditions varies. Consultation with healthcare professionals is crucial to ensure that IF aligns with individual health needs and is implemented safely and effectively. Personalized guidance can help tailor fasting approaches to accommodate specific health conditions and overall well-being.

Potential Risks and Precautions

Intermittent Fasting (IF) can offer various health benefits, but it's essential to be aware of potential risks and take precautions, especially for certain individuals or health conditions. Here are some potential risks and precautions associated with Intermittent Fasting:

- Nutrient Deficiency:
- Risk: Extended fasting periods may lead to nutrient deficiencies if not carefully planned. Insufficient intake of essential vitamins and minerals can have adverse effects on overall health.
- Precaution: Plan well-balanced meals during eating windows to ensure adequate nutrient intake.

Consider consulting with a registered dietitian for personalized advice.

- Disordered Eating Patterns:
  - Risk: IF may trigger or exacerbate disordered eating patterns in susceptible individuals. It can lead to an unhealthy preoccupation with food or an increased risk of binge eating.
  - Precaution: Individuals with a history of eating disorders or those prone to disordered eating should approach IF cautiously. Seek guidance from mental health professionals if needed.

- Impact on Hormones:
  - Risk: IF may affect hormonal balance, potentially leading to disruptions in menstrual cycles for some women. Hormonal changes can also impact mood and energy levels.
  - Precaution: Women should be mindful of any hormonal changes and consider adjusting fasting schedules if adverse effects are observed. Consultation with healthcare professionals is advisable.

- Hypoglycemia:

- Risk: Individuals with diabetes, especially those on certain medications, may be at risk of hypoglycemia (low blood sugar) during fasting periods, leading to symptoms such as dizziness and weakness.

- Precaution: Monitor blood sugar levels regularly and consult with healthcare professionals for adjustments in medication and fasting schedules. Stay hydrated to help prevent hypoglycemia.

- Dehydration:

- Risk: Fasting periods can contribute to dehydration, leading to headaches, fatigue, and other complications. Inadequate fluid intake may impact overall health.

- Precaution: Ensure proper hydration during fasting periods by drinking water and other non-caloric beverages. Be mindful of individual fluid needs, especially in different climates or during exercise.

- Electrolyte Imbalances:

- Risk: Extended fasting may lead to electrolyte imbalances, which can affect various bodily functions, including muscle contractions and nerve signaling.

- Precaution: Include electrolyte-rich foods in your diet or consider electrolyte supplements, especially during prolonged fasting. Regular hydration supports electrolyte balance.

- **Medication Interactions:**
- Risk: IF may interact with certain medications, affecting their absorption or effectiveness. Medication timing may need adjustments during fasting periods.

- Precaution: Consult with healthcare professionals to assess potential interactions and make necessary adjustments to medication schedules.

- **Adverse Effects on Sleep:**
- Risk: Irregular eating patterns or fasting too close to bedtime may disrupt sleep. Poor sleep can have a negative impact on overall health and well-being.

- Precaution: Pay attention to the timing of fasting periods, especially if you notice adverse effects on sleep. Prioritize consistent sleep schedules for optimal rest.

- Stress and Mental Health:
- Risk: For some individuals, the stress associated with strict adherence to fasting schedules may negatively impact mental health, leading to increased anxiety or irritability.
- Precaution: Maintain a flexible and balanced approach to IF. If stress or mental health concerns arise, consider adjusting fasting patterns and seek support from mental health professionals.

- Individual Variability:
- Risk: Responses to IF can vary among individuals. What works well for one person may not be suitable for another. Individual factors, such as health status and lifestyle, should be considered.
- Precaution: Be attentive to your body's signals and adjust your fasting approach based on individual responses. If in doubt, consult with healthcare professionals.

While Intermittent Fasting can offer health benefits, it's crucial to be aware of potential risks and take appropriate precautions. Individualized approaches, regular monitoring, and consultation with healthcare and nutrition professionals can help ensure that IF is implemented safely and effectively, taking into account individual health needs and goals.

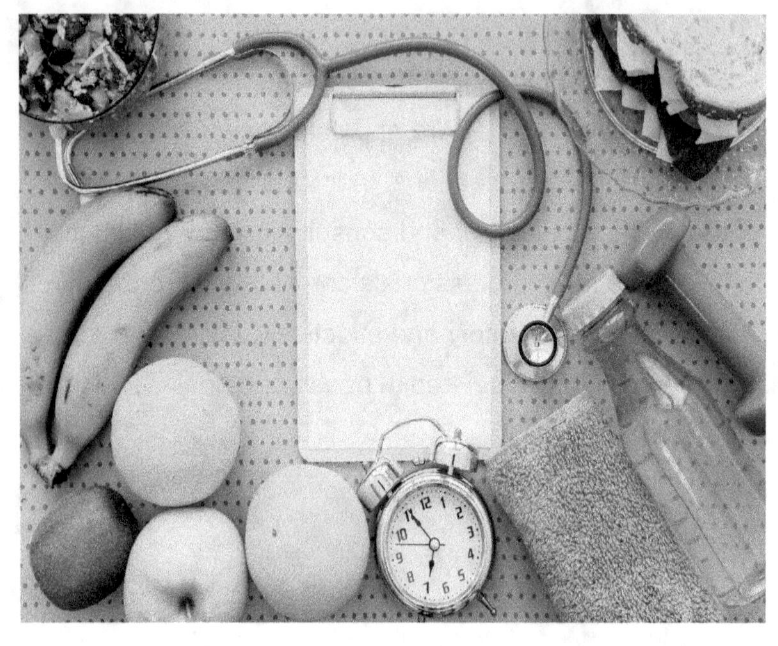

CHAPTER SIX

Intermittent Fasting for Women

Addressing Gender-Specific Considerations

Intermittent Fasting (IF) for women requires attention to gender-specific considerations due to hormonal and physiological differences. While IF can be beneficial for many women, it's crucial to approach it mindfully. Here are key considerations for women practicing Intermittent Fasting:

- Hormonal Impact:

 - Menstrual Cycle: IF may affect menstrual cycles in some women. Irregular periods or hormonal imbalances can occur, impacting fertility and overall well-being.

 - Adjustment: Consider adjusting fasting schedules based on your menstrual cycle. Some women find that a more flexible approach or shorter fasting

windows during certain phases of the cycle works
best.

- Fertility and Pregnancy:

- Impact on Fertility: Long-term or intense IF may
affect fertility in some women. It's essential to
prioritize adequate nutrient intake, especially for
those planning to conceive.

- Pregnancy: IF is generally not recommended
during pregnancy. Adequate nutrition is crucial
during this time, and any dietary changes should be
discussed with healthcare professionals.

- Bone Health:

- Concerns for Bone Density: Prolonged periods of
low-calorie intake, common in certain IF
approaches, can pose risks to bone health. Women,
particularly those at risk of osteoporosis, should
ensure sufficient calcium and vitamin D intake.

- Include Nutrient-Dense Foods: Incorporate dairy
products, leafy greens, and other calcium-rich foods
in your eating windows. Consider seeking
personalized advice from a registered dietitian.

- Energy and Performance:

- Individual Responses: Women may have different responses to fasting in terms of energy levels and exercise performance. Some may thrive, while others may experience fatigue.

- Adaptation: Allow time for your body to adapt to IF. Be attentive to energy levels and adjust fasting windows or exercise intensity accordingly.

- Stress and Cortisol Levels:

- Impact on Stress: IF may contribute to increased stress levels in some women, leading to potential hormonal imbalances. Chronic stress can affect overall health and well-being.

- Stress Management: Prioritize stress management techniques such as meditation, deep breathing, or yoga. A balanced approach to IF can help minimize stress.

- Individualized Approach:

- Variability in Responses: Responses to IF vary widely among women. Individual factors such as age, health status, and lifestyle play a role in determining the suitability of IF.

- Experiment Gradually: Start with a gradual approach to IF and monitor how your body responds. Adjust fasting windows and eating patterns based on individual comfort and well-being.

- Post-Menopausal Considerations:
- Hormonal Changes: Post-menopausal women may experience hormonal changes that impact metabolism and body composition. IF may need to be adapted to these changes.
- Focus on Nutrient-Dense Foods: Prioritize nutrient-dense foods to support overall health. Consider consulting with healthcare professionals for guidance on IF during post-menopausal years.

- Consistency vs. Flexibility:
- Adherence to Schedules: Some women may find that strict adherence to fasting schedules is challenging, especially during different phases of life.
- Flexible Approach: Consider a more flexible approach to IF, allowing for adjustments based on hormonal fluctuations, stress levels, and individual preferences.

- Hydration and Electrolytes:

 - Water Retention: Hormonal fluctuations during the menstrual cycle can lead to water retention. Staying hydrated is crucial, and balancing electrolytes can help mitigate bloating.

 - Monitor Hydration: Pay attention to hydration levels, especially during fasting periods. Include electrolyte-rich foods or consider supplements if needed.

- Consultation with Healthcare Professionals:

 - Individualized Guidance: Before starting IF, especially for women with specific health concerns or conditions, consultation with healthcare professionals is advisable. They can provide tailored advice based on an individual's health status.

Women can benefit from Intermittent Fasting, but it's essential to approach it with awareness of gender-specific considerations. Adapting fasting schedules based on menstrual cycles, prioritizing nutrient-dense foods, and being mindful of individual responses are crucial for a positive and sustainable experience with IF. Consultation with healthcare and nutrition professionals can provide personalized guidance tailored to women's unique needs and circumstances.

Hormonal Impacts

Intermittent Fasting (IF) can have varying hormonal impacts on women, and these effects may be influenced by individual factors such as age, health status, and lifestyle. Here's an overview of some hormonal considerations associated with IF for women:

- Insulin Sensitivity:

- Positive Impact: IF may enhance insulin sensitivity, helping the body respond more effectively to insulin. This can be beneficial for managing blood sugar levels and reducing the risk of insulin resistance.

- Growth Hormone (GH):

- Increased Secretion: Short-term fasting periods may lead to an increase in growth hormone secretion. GH plays a role in fat metabolism and muscle preservation.

- **Cortisol Levels:**
  - Potential Fluctuations: IF can lead to fluctuations in cortisol levels, especially during fasting periods. Cortisol is a stress hormone, and prolonged or intense fasting may contribute to increased stress.

- **Leptin and Ghrelin:**
  - Regulation of Appetite: IF may influence the regulation of appetite hormones, such as leptin and ghrelin. Changes in these hormones can impact hunger and satiety cues.

- **Estrogen and Menstrual Cycle:**
  - Menstrual Irregularities: Some women may experience changes in their menstrual cycle, including irregular periods or amenorrhea (absence of menstruation), especially with more extreme forms of fasting.
  - Adaptation: Women should pay attention to how their menstrual cycle responds to IF. Adjustments in

fasting patterns may be necessary to support hormonal balance.

- Thyroid Hormones:
- Potential Impact: Extended fasting or insufficient calorie intake may influence thyroid hormone levels. This can affect metabolism and energy production.
- Nutrient-Dense Diet: Ensure a nutrient-dense diet during eating windows to support thyroid function. Adequate intake of iodine and selenium is essential for thyroid health.

- Reproductive Hormones:
- Individual Responses: IF may have varying effects on reproductive hormones, including follicle-stimulating hormone (FSH) and luteinizing hormone (LH). Individual responses can differ.

- Adiponectin:
- Potential Increase: IF may contribute to an increase in adiponectin, a hormone associated with improved insulin sensitivity and fat metabolism.

- Post-Menopausal Hormonal Changes:

- Consideration for Hormonal Shifts:
Post-menopausal women may experience hormonal changes. IF may need to be adapted to these shifts, and maintaining bone health becomes crucial.

- Individual Variability:
- Responses Vary: Hormonal responses to IF can vary widely among women. Individual factors such as age, health status, and overall lifestyle play a role in determining these responses.

- Hormonal Adaptation:
- Allow Time for Adaptation: Hormonal adaptations to IF may take time. Women are encouraged to allow their bodies to adapt gradually and be attentive to any signs of hormonal imbalances.

- Stress Management:
- Mind-Body Practices: Given the potential impact of IF on cortisol levels, incorporating stress management practices such as meditation, deep breathing, or yoga can be beneficial.

Intermittent Fasting can influence various hormones in women, and responses are highly individualized. While some women may experience positive effects on insulin sensitivity and fat metabolism, others may face challenges such as menstrual irregularities. It's crucial for women to approach IF with awareness, be mindful of hormonal cues, and make adjustments based on individual responses. Consultation with healthcare professionals, especially for those with specific health concerns, can provide personalized guidance on incorporating IF into a woman's lifestyle in a way that supports overall health and well-being.

Intermittent Fasting for Special Populations

- Pregnant Women

Intermittent Fasting (IF) is generally not recommended for pregnant women due to the increased nutritional demands during pregnancy. Pregnancy requires a steady supply of essential nutrients for fetal development and maternal well-being. IF involves extended periods of fasting, potentially leading to inadequate calorie and nutrient intake, which can pose risks to both the mother and the developing fetus. Pregnant women need sufficient energy, vitamins, and minerals to support the growth of the baby and maintain their own health.

Restricting food intake through fasting may result in nutrient deficiencies, impacting fetal development and increasing the risk of complications. Additionally, fasting could lead to fluctuations in blood sugar levels and energy levels, potentially affecting the overall well-being of the pregnant woman.

It is crucial for pregnant women to prioritize a well-balanced and nutrient-dense diet throughout their pregnancy. Any dietary changes or fasting practices during pregnancy should be discussed with healthcare professionals to ensure the health and safety of both the mother and the baby. Pregnant women should focus on maintaining adequate nutrition, staying hydrated, and following a balanced eating pattern recommended by healthcare providers.

- Athletes

Intermittent Fasting (IF) among athletes is a nuanced practice that requires careful consideration of individual training demands, performance goals, and overall well-being. Athletes engaging in IF should approach it with awareness of potential effects on training adaptations, recovery, and energy levels.

For endurance athletes, IF might affect glycogen stores and performance during prolonged activities. Strategic planning of fasting periods, such as aligning them with rest days, can help mitigate potential impacts on endurance training. Resistance training athletes may find IF compatible with muscle building, provided protein intake is prioritized during eating windows to support recovery and muscle synthesis.

Hydration becomes paramount during fasting periods to prevent dehydration, particularly for athletes who engage in intense training. Electrolyte balance should also be maintained, and athletes must monitor their energy levels to avoid compromising performance.

Timing of fasting windows is crucial for athletes to ensure adequate fuel for workouts. Some athletes may benefit from adjusting fasting schedules to align with training sessions, allowing for pre- and post-workout nutrition.

Individual responses to IF vary, and athletes should monitor their performance, recovery, and overall well-being. Athletes with specific dietary requirements, such as those with higher calorie needs, should ensure sufficient intake during eating windows to meet their energy demands.

Consultation with sports nutrition professionals or dietitians can provide personalized guidance. Athletes should prioritize nutrient-dense foods during eating windows, emphasizing a well-balanced diet to meet their macro- and micronutrient needs.

In summary, IF can be compatible with athletic training when approached thoughtfully. Athletes should tailor fasting strategies to their specific sport, training schedule, and individual responses. Professional guidance, careful monitoring of performance metrics, and attention to nutritional needs are essential for integrating IF into an athlete's routine while maintaining optimal physical performance and well-being.

Individuals with Health Conditions

Intermittent Fasting (IF) for individuals with health conditions requires a cautious and individualized approach. While IF has shown potential benefits, it's crucial for those with specific health concerns to consult healthcare professionals before adopting any fasting regimen.

- Diabetes:

- Risk of Hypoglycemia: Individuals with diabetes should carefully consider IF, as fasting periods may lead to fluctuations in blood sugar levels. Medication adjustments and close monitoring are essential to prevent hypoglycemia.

- **Cardiovascular Conditions:**
- Potential Benefits: IF may offer cardiovascular benefits, but those with heart conditions should consult healthcare professionals. IF might impact blood pressure and cholesterol levels, necessitating personalized guidance.

- **Gastrointestinal Disorders:**
- Varied Responses: Individuals with gastrointestinal conditions may experience varied responses to IF. Some may find relief, while others may face challenges such as exacerbation of symptoms. Professional guidance is crucial.

- **Eating Disorders:**
- Caution Advised: Those with a history of eating disorders should approach IF cautiously. Fasting practices can trigger or worsen disordered eating patterns. Mental health professionals should be involved in the decision-making process.

- Thyroid Disorders:

- Impact on Thyroid Function: IF may influence thyroid hormone levels, potentially affecting those with thyroid disorders. Regular monitoring and consultation with healthcare professionals are necessary.

- Autoimmune Conditions:

- Inflammatory Response: IF's impact on inflammation may be relevant for individuals with autoimmune conditions. Close monitoring and collaboration with healthcare providers are crucial to assess responses.

- Neurological Disorders:

- Potential Neuroprotective Effects: Some research suggests potential neuroprotective effects of IF. However, its application for individuals with neurological disorders requires careful consideration and monitoring.

- Pregnancy and Lactation:

- Not Recommended: IF is generally not recommended during pregnancy and lactation. Adequate nutrition is crucial during these periods, and any dietary changes should be discussed with healthcare professionals.

- Medication Interaction:
- Adjustments may be Needed: IF may interact with certain medications. Individuals on medication regimens should consult with healthcare professionals to ensure proper management and dosing.

- Individualized Approach:
- Consultation is Key: Before embarking on IF, individuals with health conditions should undergo a comprehensive health assessment. Consultation with healthcare professionals, including dietitians and specialists, is essential for personalized advice.

In conclusion, IF can have varied impacts on individuals with health conditions. While it may offer benefits, it requires careful consideration and individualized planning. Collaboration with healthcare professionals is paramount to ensure that IF aligns with individual health needs, medications, and overall well-being. Professional guidance helps mitigate potential risks and maximizes the potential benefits for those with specific health concerns.

CHAPTER SEVEN

Recipes and Meal Ideas

Creating delicious and nutritious meals is essential for those practicing intermittent fasting. Optimal recipes focus on nutrient-dense ingredients and a balanced combination of proteins, healthy fats, and complex carbohydrates to support energy levels during eating windows.

Start your day with a protein-rich breakfast like a Mediterranean-style omelette filled with tomatoes, spinach, and feta cheese. For lunch, consider a hearty salad with grilled salmon or a vegetarian

Buddha bowl featuring quinoa, roasted sweet potatoes, and chickpeas. A chicken and vegetable stir-fry with a flavorful soy-ginger sauce makes for a satisfying dinner option.

Simple and quick recipes like an egg and avocado wrap or a Greek yogurt parfait can be enjoyed as snacks between fasting periods. For a refreshing option, blend a smoothie bowl with frozen berries, banana, and spinach, topped with granola and nuts.

Experiment with flavors by trying recipes like quinoa-stuffed bell peppers or turkey and vegetable lettuce wraps. Cap off the day with a light but flavorful option like caprese skewers with cherry tomatoes, mozzarella balls, and fresh basil drizzled with balsamic glaze.

These meal ideas offer variety and flexibility while meeting the nutritional needs of individuals practicing intermittent fasting. Adjusting portion sizes and ingredients based on personal preferences ensures a delicious and satisfying experience while supporting overall health and well-being.

Fasting-Friendly Recipes

Fasting-friendly recipes should focus on nutrient-dense, satisfying options to support energy levels during eating windows. Here are a few ideas:

- Grilled Salmon Salad:
  - Ingredients: Grilled salmon, mixed greens, cherry tomatoes, cucumber, avocado.
  - Dressing: olive oil, lemon juice, salt, and pepper.
  - Instructions: Combine salad ingredients, top with grilled salmon. Drizzle with dressing.

- Vegetarian Buddha Bowl:
  - Ingredients: Quinoa, roasted sweet potatoes, chickpeas, spinach, cherry tomatoes.
  - Sauce: Tahini, lemon juice, garlic, salt.
  - Instructions: Arrange ingredients in a bowl. Drizzle with tahini sauce.

- Chicken and Vegetable Stir-Fry:

- Ingredients: Chicken breast, broccoli, bell peppers, snap peas.

Soy sauce, ginger, garlic, and sesame oil make up the sauce.

- Instructions: Stir-fry chicken and vegetables. Add sauce, cook until tender.

- Egg Avocado Wrap:

- Ingredients: Scrambled eggs, avocado slices, whole-grain wrap.

- Add-ons: Spinach, cherry tomatoes.

- Instructions: Fill the wrap with scrambled eggs, avocado, and veggies.

- Mediterranean Chickpea Salad:

- Ingredients: Chickpeas, cherry tomatoes, cucumber, red onion, feta cheese, olives.

- Dressing: Olive oil, red wine vinegar, oregano, salt, and pepper.

- Instructions: Combine salad ingredients. Toss with dressing.

- Greek Yogurt Parfait:

- Ingredients: - Greek yogurt, mixed berries, granola, and honey.

- Instructions: Layer yogurt, berries, and granola. Drizzle with honey.

- Quinoa Stuffed Bell Peppers:

- Ingredients: Quinoa, black beans, corn, diced tomatoes, bell peppers.

- Seasoning: Cumin, chili powder, garlic powder.

- Instructions: Mix ingredients, stuff peppers, bake until peppers are tender.

- Turkey and Vegetable Lettuce Wraps:

- Ingredients: Ground turkey, lettuce leaves, diced bell peppers, carrots, and cucumber.

- Sauce: Hoisin sauce, soy sauce, ginger.

- Instructions: Cook turkey, add veggies, and sauce. Spoon into lettuce leaves.

- Smoothie Bowl:

- Ingredients: Frozen berries, banana, spinach, almond milk.

- - Toppings include granola, chopped almonds, and chia seeds.

- Instructions: Blend ingredients, top with granola and nuts.

- Caprese Skewers:

- Ingredients: Cherry tomatoes, mozzarella balls, fresh basil leaves.

- Dressing: Balsamic glaze.

- Instructions: Thread tomatoes, mozzarella, and basil onto skewers. Drizzle with balsamic glaze.

These recipes provide a balance of proteins, healthy fats, and complex carbohydrates, making them suitable for individuals practicing intermittent fasting. Adjust portion sizes and ingredients based on personal preferences and dietary needs.

Tracking Progress and Adjusting

Tracking progress and adjusting in the context of intermittent fasting (IF) involves a mindful and dynamic approach to ensure the effectiveness and sustainability of the fasting routine. Regularly monitoring key health metrics such as body weight, composition, blood sugar levels, and energy performance provides valuable insights into the impact of IF on individual well-being. Adjustments can then be made to fasting schedules, meal compositions, or exercise routines based on these observations.

For optimal results, individuals should pay attention to their body's responses, including hormonal balance, nutrient intake, and digestive health. Women, in particular, may need to adapt their fasting schedules based on menstrual cycles. The significance of regular consultations with healthcare professionals, nutritionists, or fitness experts cannot be overstated, providing personalized guidance for making informed adjustments.

Mindful self-reflection, sleep quality monitoring, and stress level observations contribute to a holistic understanding of the individual's response to IF. This iterative process allows individuals to fine-tune their fasting protocols, ensuring that IF aligns with their health goals and enhances overall well-being. The combination of proactive tracking and thoughtful adjustments forms the cornerstone of a successful and sustainable intermittent fasting journey.

Monitoring Health Metrics

Monitoring health metrics is a crucial aspect of any wellness journey, providing valuable insights into one's physical well-being and the effectiveness of lifestyle choices. In the context of intermittent fasting (IF), tracking specific health metrics helps individuals tailor their approach for optimal results.

- Body Weight and Composition:

- Tracking: Regularly measuring body weight and assessing changes in fat mass and lean muscle mass.

- Importance: Offers a quantitative view of progress and informs adjustments to fasting schedules or dietary choices.

- Blood Sugar Levels:

- Tracking: Regular monitoring, especially for individuals with diabetes or those concerned about blood sugar regulation.

- Importance: Guides adjustments to fasting windows and meal composition, ensuring stable blood sugar levels.

- Energy Levels and Performance:

- Tracking: Paying attention to energy levels, exercise performance, and overall vitality.

- Importance: Indicates how well the fasting routine aligns with energy demands and may prompt adjustments to optimize physical performance.

- Hormonal Balance:

- Tracking: Particularly relevant for women monitoring menstrual cycles and hormonal responses.

- Importance: Helps adapt fasting schedules to support hormonal balance and overall well-being.

- **Nutrient Intake:**

- Tracking: Recording nutrient intake, ensuring sufficient macro- and micronutrients.

- Importance: Informs dietary adjustments, ensuring nutritional needs are met during eating windows.

- **Sleep Quality and Stress Levels:**

- Tracking: Observing sleep patterns and stress levels during fasting periods.

- Importance: Guides adjustments to fasting or eating times to support better sleep and stress management.

- **Digestive Health:**

- Tracking: Monitoring digestive comfort and regularity.

- Importance: Helps adapt dietary fiber intake or hydration levels to support optimal digestive health.

Consistent tracking of these health metrics empowers individuals practicing intermittent fasting to make informed decisions, allowing for a personalized and effective approach to health and well-being. Regular assessment and adjustments based on these metrics contribute to a sustainable and positive intermittent fasting experience.

Fine-Tuning Fasting Plans

Fine-tuning fasting plans is a key aspect of optimizing the effectiveness and sustainability of intermittent fasting (IF). As individuals progress on their IF journey, they may need to make adjustments based on their evolving goals, preferences, and health responses. Here are essential considerations for fine-tuning fasting plans:

- Fasting Windows:

- Observation: Assess how the current fasting window aligns with energy levels, daily schedule, and lifestyle.

- Adjustment: Gradually modify fasting durations, experimenting with shorter or longer windows to find the most sustainable approach.

- Meal Composition:

- Observation: Monitor the nutrient density of meals during eating windows.

- Adjustment: Optimize the balance of proteins, fats, and carbohydrates to meet individual nutritional needs and support overall well-being.

- Exercise Timing:

- Observation: Evaluate the timing of exercise sessions in relation to fasting and eating periods.

- Adjustment: Experiment with different exercise timings to enhance performance and recovery, ensuring it complements fasting goals.

- Hydration Strategies:

- Observation: Pay attention to hydration levels, especially during fasting periods.

- Adjustment: Fine-tune water intake, considering factors like climate, activity levels, and individual hydration needs.

- **Supplementation:**

- Observation: Assess whether nutrient deficiencies or specific health goals necessitate supplementation.

- Adjustment: Consult with healthcare professionals to incorporate targeted supplements that complement the fasting plan.

- **Cyclical Fasting:**

- Observation: Consider implementing periodic variations in fasting patterns.

- Adjustment: Experiment with cyclical fasting, such as alternate-day fasting or periodic longer fasts, to explore different metabolic responses.

- **Social Considerations:**

- Observation: Reflect on how fasting aligns with social situations and personal relationships.

- Adjustment: Plan flexible fasting schedules to accommodate social events, ensuring IF remains adaptable to various lifestyle scenarios.

- **Listening to Body Signals:**
- Observation: Be attuned to hunger cues, energy levels, and overall well-being.
- Adjustment: Adjust fasting plans based on individual responses, allowing flexibility for intuitive adjustments when needed.

- **Consistent Monitoring:**
- Observation: Continuously monitor health metrics and progress.
- Adjustment: Regularly review tracking data and make data-informed adjustments to ensure sustained progress and well-being.

Fine-tuning fasting plans is a personalized and iterative process that requires attention to individual responses and goals. Regular self-assessment, coupled with an openness to experiment and adjust, ensures that intermittent fasting remains an adaptable and beneficial lifestyle approach over the long term. Consulting with healthcare professionals or nutrition experts can provide valuable guidance in the fine-tuning process.

FAQs and Common Misconceptions

Addressing Frequently Asked Questions

FAQs (Frequently Asked Questions) and Common Misconceptions about Intermittent Fasting (IF):

1. Can I Drink Water During Fasting?
   - Yes. Staying hydrated is crucial during fasting. Water, herbal teas, and black coffee are generally allowed. However, sugary drinks or those with added calories may break the fast.

2. Will Intermittent Fasting Slow Down My Metabolism?

- No. IF can actually support metabolism by promoting fat utilization. It's essential to maintain a balanced diet during eating windows to prevent metabolic slowdown.

3. Is IF Suitable for Everyone?

- Not necessarily. Individuals with certain health conditions, pregnant or breastfeeding women, and those with a history of eating disorders should consult healthcare professionals before starting IF.

4. Do I Need to Count Calories during IF?

- It depends. While some find success without counting, others may benefit from tracking calories to ensure adequate intake during eating windows, especially if weight management is a goal.

5. Will IF Lead to Muscle Loss?

- Not if done right. Proper protein intake and resistance training can help preserve lean muscle mass during IF. Nutrient-dense meals are essential.

6. Can I Exercise While Fasting?

- Yes. Many people exercise during fasting, and some even prefer it. Adjusting the timing of workouts within eating windows can optimize energy levels and recovery.

7. Does IF Affect Hormones?

- Yes. IF can influence hormones like insulin, growth hormone, and cortisol. It's essential to understand individual responses and consider hormonal factors, especially for women.

8. Will IF Lead to Nutrient Deficiencies?

- Possibly. Monitoring nutrient intake is crucial. A well-balanced diet during eating windows and, if necessary, supplementation can help prevent deficiencies.

9. Can I Follow IF Long-Term?

- It depends on the individual. Some people find IF sustainable long-term, while others may prefer intermittent periods of fasting. Consistency and individual adaptation are key.

10. Is Skipping Breakfast Unhealthy?

- Not necessarily. Skipping breakfast as part of IF doesn't inherently make it unhealthy. What matters is overall nutrient intake and meal quality during eating windows.

Common Misconceptions:

1. IF is a One-Size-Fits-All Approach:
   - Reality: IF should be tailored to individual needs and goals. What works for one person might not work for the next.

2. IF Guarantees Weight Loss:
   - Reality: While IF can aid weight loss for many, individual results vary. Consistent overall lifestyle factors, including diet and exercise, play crucial roles.

3. IF is a Quick Fix:
   - Reality: IF is a lifestyle approach, not a quick fix. Sustainable results require consistency, patience, and a holistic approach to health.

4. IF Doesn't Require Nutrient Consideration:

- Reality: Nutrient-dense meals are crucial during eating windows to ensure overall health. Ignoring nutrient intake can lead to deficiencies.

5. IF Negatively Impacts Women:
   - Reality: While some women thrive with IF, others may experience hormonal imbalances. Women should adapt fasting plans to their individual needs and consult healthcare professionals.

In Summary:

Intermittent Fasting is a versatile approach, but it requires thoughtful consideration. Addressing FAQs and dispelling misconceptions helps individuals navigate IF more effectively, fostering a balanced and informed approach to their health and well-being. Always consult healthcare professionals for personalized advice.

Dispelling Myths Surrounding Intermittent Fasting

1. Myth: Intermittent Fasting Slows Down Metabolism:

- Reality: IF can support metabolism by promoting fat utilization. However, it's crucial to maintain a balanced diet during eating windows to prevent metabolic slowdown.

2. Myth: Skipping Breakfast is Always Unhealthy:
   - Reality: IF often involves skipping breakfast, but it doesn't inherently make it unhealthy. The focus should be on overall nutrient intake and meal quality during eating windows.

3. Myth: Intermittent Fasting Leads to Muscle Loss:
   - Reality: When done right, with proper protein intake and resistance training, IF can help preserve lean muscle mass.

4. Myth: Intermittent fasting is only used to lose weight:
   - Reality: While IF can aid weight loss, it offers various health benefits beyond weight management, including metabolic flexibility and improved cellular health.

5. Myth: Intermittent Fasting Works the Same for Everyone:

   - Reality: IF is a personalized approach. What works for one person might not work for the next. Individual factors such as health conditions and lifestyle should be considered.

6. Myth: Intermittent Fasting Causes Nutrient Deficiencies:

   - Reality: Monitoring nutrient intake is crucial during IF. A well-balanced diet during eating windows and, if necessary, supplementation can prevent deficiencies.

7. Myth: Intermittent Fasting is a Quick Fix:

   - Reality: IF is a lifestyle approach, not a quick fix. Sustainable results require consistency, patience, and overall healthy habits.

8. Myth: Intermittent Fasting Negatively Impacts Women:

   - Reality: While some women thrive with IF, others may experience hormonal imbalances. Women

should adapt fasting plans to their individual needs
and consult healthcare professionals.

9. Myth: Intermittent Fasting Means No Exercise:
   - Reality: Many people exercise during fasting,
and some even prefer it. Adjusting the timing of
workouts within eating windows can optimize energy
levels and recovery.

10. Myth: Intermittent Fasting Guarantees
Long-Term Success:
   - Reality: Long-term success with IF depends on
individual factors, adaptability, and overall lifestyle
choices. It is not a foolproof solution for everyone.

Dispelling myths surrounding intermittent fasting is
crucial for promoting a nuanced and informed
understanding of this lifestyle approach.
Acknowledging its diverse effects on individuals and
clarifying misconceptions ensures that people can
adopt intermittent fasting with realistic expectations
and personalized strategies for their health and
well-being. Seek expert help for individualized
advice.

Conclusion

In conclusion, Intermittent Fasting (IF) has emerged as a popular and versatile approach to health and well-being, challenging traditional notions about meal timing and frequency. With its roots in ancient practices and a growing body of contemporary research, IF has gained recognition for its potential benefits, including weight management, improved metabolic health, and cellular rejuvenation.

The flexibility inherent in IF allows individuals to choose from various fasting protocols, such as time-restricted eating, alternate-day fasting, or periodic extended fasts, making it adaptable to diverse lifestyles. However, it is essential to approach IF with a nuanced understanding, recognizing that what works for one person may not be suitable for another. Individual factors, such as health conditions, hormonal balance, and personal preferences, should be carefully considered.

Dispelling myths surrounding IF is crucial for fostering informed decision-making. Contrary to misconceptions, IF, when done appropriately, does not inherently slow down metabolism, cause muscle loss, or negatively impact women. It is not a one-size-fits-all solution, and its effectiveness depends on factors like consistency, overall diet quality, and lifestyle choices.

The journey with IF requires ongoing self-assessment, tracking progress, and making adjustments based on individual responses. Whether one seeks weight management, improved energy levels, or metabolic flexibility, IF can be a valuable tool when integrated into a holistic approach to health, including regular exercise, mindful eating, and sufficient hydration.

As individuals embark on their intermittent fasting journey, it is crucial to approach it with realistic expectations and consult with healthcare professionals or nutrition experts for personalized guidance. IF's potential benefits are diverse, but the key to long-term success lies in a balanced and sustainable approach, where health and well-being remain at the forefront.